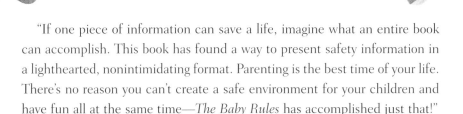

What People Are Saying About The Baby Rules

"If one piece of information can save a life, imagine what an entire book can accomplish. This book has found a way to present safety information in a lighthearted, nonintimidating format. Parenting is the best time of your life. There's no reason you can't create a safe environment for your children and have fun all at the same time—*The Baby Rules* has accomplished just that!"

Ann Brown
Former chairman of the U.S. Consumer Product Safety Commission

"*The Baby Rules* is an excellent resource for new and 'seasoned' parents alike. Seeing the world from the child's perspective is just what the National SAFE KIDS Campaign recommends!"

Heather Paul, Ph.D.
Executive director, National SAFE KIDS Campaign

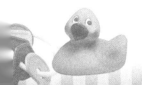

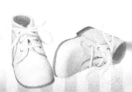

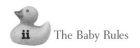 The Baby Rules

"A surprisingly upbeat, funny and captivating look at vaccines. Through the eyes of a child, the authors make a difficult, and often sobering topic, engaging."

Paul A. Offit, M.D.
Director, Vaccine Education Center
The Children's Hospital of Philadelphia
Professor of Pediatrics
The University of Pennsylvania School of Medicine

"This book [helps] raise the awareness of parents and other adults about the safety of children. I am especially pleased that the authors included information about the importance of providing a safe play environment. Both of these factors put adults on notice to protect our most precious commodity—children."

Donna Thompson, Ph.D.
Director, National Program for Playground Safety

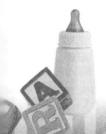
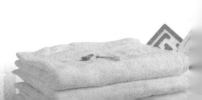

"Thank you for sharing your book with me. I found it easy to read, and a quick guide to what new parents need to know about their newborns."

Michael Lewis, Ph.D.
University distinguished professor of Pediatrics and Psychiatry, Robert Wood Johnson Medical School, and author of *Altering Fate: Why the Past Does Not Predict the Future*

"As the mother of six children, I have learned that while practical information is important, maintaining a sense of humor is essential in raising children safely in an often-scary world. Nothing is more natural than breastfeeding a baby, but the process is learned, not instinctive. Since babies don't come with instruction manuals, *The Baby Rules* includes lots of valuable information in a humorous and understandable format, and I am pleased that the author included information about breastfeeding—the best way to get babies off to a healthy start in life."

Anne Smith, BA, IBCLC, RLC
International board-certified lactation consultant
www.breastfeedingbasics.com

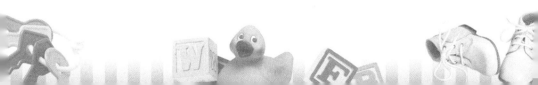

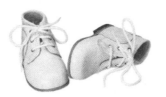

The
BABY RULES

The Insider's Guide
to Raising Your Parents

Jamie Schaefer-Wilson
Jo Anne Germinario

Health Communications, Inc.
Deerfield Beach, Florida

www.hcibooks.com

Library of Congress Cataloging-in-Publication Data

Schaefer-Wilson, Jamie, 1969–
    The baby rules : the insider's guide to raising your parents / Jamie
Schaefer-Wilson, Jo Anne Germinario.
        p. cm.
    ISBN 0-7573-0198-3
    i. Infants—Care.   2. Mother and infant.   3. Safety education.
I. Germinario, Jo Anne.   II. Title.

HQ774.S35 2004
649'.122—dc22

                                                                    2003067635

Publisher: Health Communications, Inc.
            3201 S.W. 15th Street
            Deerfield Beach, FL 33442-8190

Cover photos ©PhotoDisc and ©Hemera Photo-Objects
Cover design by Lawna Patterson Oldfield
Inside book design by Larissa Hise Henoch
Inside book formatting by Dawn Von Strolley Grove

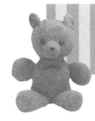

Contents

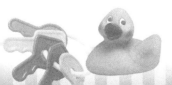

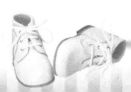

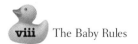

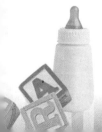

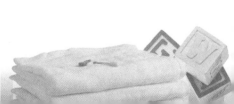

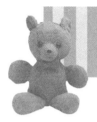

Foreword

For many years I was known as the mother of children's safety and now I'm the grandmother. I have spent much of my life fighting for safe environments: I spent eight years as the Chairman of the U.S. Consumer Product Safety Commission and thirty years as a children's safety survey specialist. Therefore, I want to make sure a book like this spotlighting safety is given the attention it deserves. While most parents think no harm will come to their children, on average every year, two and a half million children are injured or killed by hazards in the home.

One piece of information can save a child's life. I sincerely believe that premise. It takes knowledge to prevent the unthinkable. But where do parents and caregivers find this knowledge? How can you

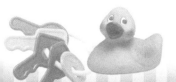

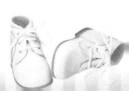

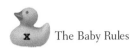

be sure that you're doing everything possible to protect your children? One step in the right direction is to arm yourself with as much information as you can about your children's environment. While you want to raise your children in a loving environment, it also needs to be a safe one.

Throughout my tenure I have heard many heart-wrenching stories of accidents in and outside of the home. For example, parents love to decorate their children's rooms with every toy and every product imaginable, but how do they know these items are safe? And it's not just about buying a safe product; it's also knowing where to place that product within a room so that it doesn't pose a danger. It's about baby-proofing the house from floor to ceiling so when an accident does happen, a tragedy doesn't follow.

My job was to ensure that as many people as possible had information that could save their child's life. This included everything from safety information to recall announcements. Although this information is readily available, it's something that needs to be checked on a daily basis. If you miss the news just once you can miss a life-threatening recall announcement. You need to know how to check this information and to be aware of the hazards in your child's environment.

The Baby Rules is a perfect primer for new or expectant parents or caregivers. Written from the perspective of babies, it presents indispensable information in a lighthearted way. After reading the book, you will feel empowered instead of insecure in your new role. Parenting should be the best time of your life, and this book helps to make it so by giving you the confidence in knowing you've done everything in your power to protect your child.

Ann Brown

Former Chairman, U.S. Consumer Product Safety Commission

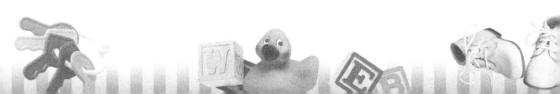

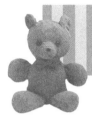

Acknowledgments

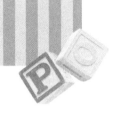

T hank you to the following people for all of your help and assistance: Ann Brown, Former Chairman, U.S. Consumer Product Safety Commission.

Dr. Paul Offit, Director, Vaccine Education Center at The Children's Hospital of Philadelphia at *www.vaccine.chop.edu*.

Bonnie Offit, M.D., Kids First, Haverford, Pennsylvania.

Donna Thompson, Ph.D., Director, National Program for Playground Safety.

Anne Smith, international board-certified lactation consultant, *Breastfeeding Basics*.

Cydney Rachel Wilson and Olivia, Michelle and Anthony Germinario, for teaching us how to be mommies, and helping us write this book.

Steven Wilson and Anthony Germinario, for all of their love and support and for being such wonderful husbands and daddies.

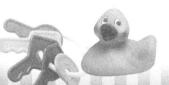

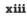

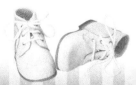

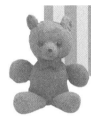
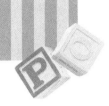

Introduction

As a TV producer, I have produced numerous segments about baby safety and I thought I was well-prepared for impending motherhood. However, once I became a new mom, I found myself an anxious, sometimes confused traveler on the bumpy but beautiful road of parenthood. I quickly learned that no matter how much you know about keeping your baby safe, sometimes it's not enough.

I personally have had three incidents with unsafe high chairs. Each incident was either in a restaurant or someone else's home. In one incident in a restaurant, the high chair was impossible to open and something in my gut said, "This isn't right." I should have listened to my instinct. As soon as I put my daughter in it and turned to sit down, the high chair started to collapse with my daughter in it. Neither my husband nor I could get the chair back

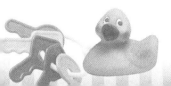

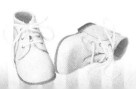

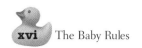

open. My husband held my daughter as I tried to pry the chair open with the waiter trying to help. A few very harrowing moments could have ended so much worse. I now listen to my mother's intuition at every turn and I watch every environment I bring my daughter into.

Unfortunately, I have met other parents who have lost children to antique cribs, unfastened TVs, car seats that were installed incorrectly and even old tree limbs that fell. My heart broke each time I heard of a child lost to a tragic and preventable accident and it became my mission to compile a book of safety information.

As a first-time mother myself, I felt I needed a parenting book that was informative yet easy to read given the time constraints on me as a new parent. As I started my journey to write this book, I discovered one disturbing fact: Some places we go to for parenting advice are unknowingly giving dangerous information to parents.

I knew something had to be done that hadn't been done in the past and that I had to add as many relevant safety tips as possible. I wanted to create a book full of tips that a parent could easily remember when placing a baby in a situation that could have potential dangers.

I was fortunate to be able to enlist the help of my close friend

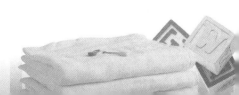

and fellow TV producer Jo Anne Germinario, who has three children of her own. Jo Anne actually unwittingly gave me the spark that started *The Baby Rules*. One day I asked her why my daughter, Cydney, was hysterical after bath time and Jo Anne looked at me and said, "Don't you know what she's saying? She's saying, 'Mommy, I'm cold, I'm cold, I'm cold.'" From that one sentence *The Baby Rules* was born. We decided to create a parenting book from the voice that hadn't yet been heard from: the baby.

We have given the voice our own interpretation and hope we have included the hearts and minds of all babies. No one can tell you for certain what will work for your own baby, as each baby is different. We can only give you some information to guide you along your journey.

Whether you follow these tips as they are presented or you tweak them to work for you, two things are certain: You will find an inner voice for your own baby and you will have learned at least one thing in this book that could save your child's life.

Enjoy your journey. May it be safe and may it be a joyful time for you, your family and your baby.

Jamie Schaefer-Wilson

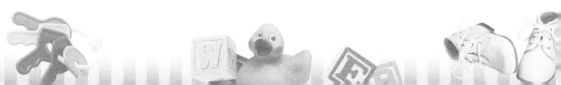

I'm Here:
At the Hospital

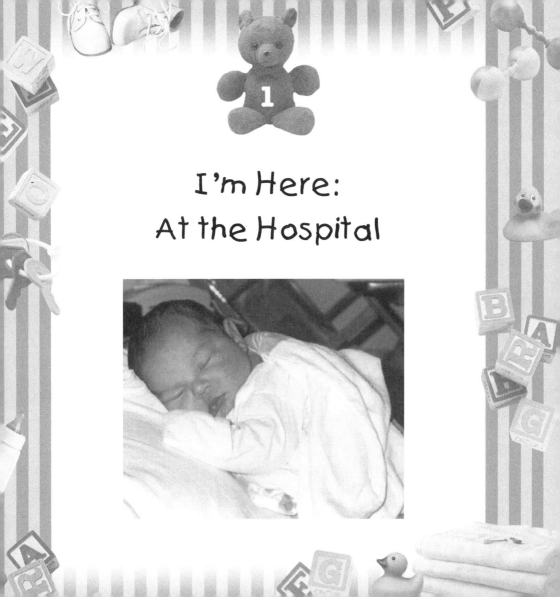

Of course you've packed your bag ahead of time, but did you remember the following: PJ's, sweats or clothes to relax in, socks, a nursing bra, a comfortable outfit for taking me home, and most of all—a robe and slippers? You'll want to be comfortable when you visit me in the nursery.

You and your doctor should have come up with a birth plan for the hospital. You did that, didn't you? Bring copies to the hospital for the nurses so everyone knows your wishes.

I hope you made a checklist to remind you what you'll need at the hospital. If you didn't, see the list on page 13. Daddy can't be running out to partake in some last-minute shopping because who only knows what he'll bring back. Besides, you're going to need his help at the hospital. If you plan ahead, you'll find it easier to relax and enjoy the moment. Remember that anything you've forgotten isn't nearly as important as just enjoying the miracle of my arrival.

 I hope you remembered to bring some lotions and shampoo. You can't pamper me if you don't pamper yourself. This isn't a hotel; it's a hospital so you need to bring any items that would make you feel at home, like some relaxing music and maybe a pen and paper to begin my baby journal.

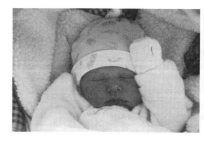

Did you bring a warm outfit for me, and my hat and booties? Keep in mind, no matter how hot or cold it is, I've never been outside before (of the womb or the hospital!).

Don't forget some goodies for the nurses. You won't want to start searching through the phone book for a good bakery or a store nearby. You will want to do something nice for them as they take care of both Mommy and me twenty-four hours a day. Doing something nice for them will put a smile on their faces. Remember that it's their faces I'll see as well as yours throughout the day.

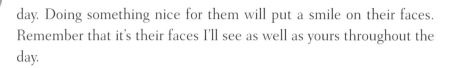 Okay, so my head is shaped like a cone and is a little shriveled. You may think I look funny, but you should see how you look to me. It wasn't easy for me to make my appearance in this world. Give me— and my head—some time to adjust.

I'm changing by the hour so take plenty of pictures please; but don't use a flash while taking photographs of me. I can't focus yet and all I see are spots. From my first day of life to my second day, I've actually doubled in age. How often can you say that? I'm ready for my close-up.

I may have just arrived in this world, but I'm hungry! I know I'm supposed to have a sucking instinct but I may need some help getting started. If you rub my cheek it may help me to begin sucking on your breast or a bottle. Even though I want to eat you may need to help teach me how it's done.

Note to grown-ups: You need to rub the side of the cheek closest to the breast I will turn toward. If you rub the wrong side, I will turn away and you'll think I'm refusing your breast, which I'm not.

If the nurse asks if you want me to spend the night in the nursery, don't feel guilty about saying, "Yes!" It's okay if the nurses take care of me during the nights at the hospital. You're probably exhausted from trying to bring me into this world and I'm going to need your full attention when we get home.

Note to grown-ups: If you're breastfeeding me, you will want to tell the nurses to bring me to your room for feedings. When debating where I'll spend my first night in this world, keep in mind that if I room in with you it will make breastfeeding easier. You held me twenty-four hours a day for nine months. I'm used to being with you!

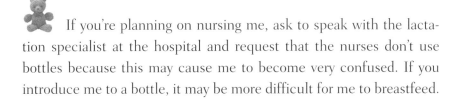 If you're planning on nursing me, ask to speak with the lactation specialist at the hospital and request that the nurses don't use bottles because this may cause me to become very confused. If you introduce me to a bottle, it may be more difficult for me to breastfeed.

Let me tell you about something that makes me feel very comfortable. . . . It's called swaddling. These hospital nurses are sooo good at it! Ask them how it's done. It's very comforting to me. If done correctly I should look like a baby burrito.

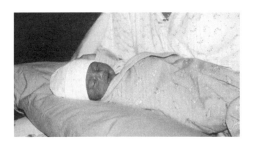

It's time for Swaddling 101. Put a square receiving blanket down like a diamond. Place me in the middle of the diamond, with my hands down at my sides. Cross the left side over me so it covers

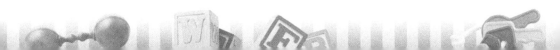

my chest and then pull the middle up and over my toes. Cross the right side around my back and under me. Don't be discouraged if I come undone—I may be a wiggly baby.

Hey, I can't stop crying. I'm wet and I'm hungry and I'm tired, too. I think Mommy or Daddy can help me but I'm having a moment right now. I know taking care of me may be harder than you thought but once we establish a routine and you figure out my needs it will become easier.

Weary, weak, worn-out. Does that describe how you feel? It's okay to be tired; you've been through a lot. That's why you have to take every opportunity to get a few moments of shut-eye. You'll feel much better once you catch up on your sleep. I tend to get a little cranky myself when I'm tired. I know it's hard to believe but it's true.

The first time you hold me—and for the first few months— you have to hold my head. I can't support my head yet, and you have to help me until I can help myself.

Please make sure all my visitors wash their hands before holding or touching me. Do you know the last time they washed those hands? I don't, and I'm very susceptible to germs. You can't be too careful. Germs spread through talking, hand-to-hand contact and sneezing. You don't need to go overboard, but you do need to be careful. I will be less susceptible when I'm over two months old. You just need to be cautious until then.

Don't fill out the birth certificate form until you are 100 percent sure of my name. Do you know what it would be like to try to change that thing? You don't have time for that kind of paperwork. I'm occupying every moment of your life and I like it. Think twice before you name me because some names can lead to an awful lot of teasing on the playground.

Bring an extra bag (or two) for the free supplies the hospital will give you. Take all of the extra diapers and formula home with you. Believe me, you'll need them! Don't be shy about this. The hospital provides you with extra goodies and I don't think either mommies or daddies want to be running to the store in the middle of the night for extra supplies. Aren't you tired enough?

Many hospitals provide disposable pads for you to change me on. These are the best! Take some of these home with you. . . . It will mean less laundry for you.

Save the hospital tags for my baby book, especially the "It's a Boy/Girl" card, and the hat I wore in the hospital, too. Always be on the lookout for keepsake opportunities, especially the free ones.

Mommies aren't going to be able to lift much the day we leave the hospital and Daddy only has two arms (like me) so have a plan for how you are getting me home. Arrange ahead of time for a family member or close friend to help us out. The more the merrier! Besides, you should probably get used to asking for extra help.

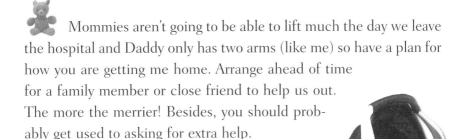

Don't forget to bring the car seat to the hospital . . . It's the law! They won't let you take me home without it and I want to get out of this place!

Note: See the car seat section of this book for how to install the seat and buckle me in!

Even if it's warm outside, bring one of my new blankets with you. I love to be snugly, and I'm not used to the change in temperature just yet.

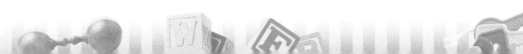

I can't see very far for the first several weeks of my life. As a matter of fact, I can only see things that are about twelve inches from my face so please try to hold things where I can see them. I want stimulation but it doesn't help if you are the only one who is stimulated.

Note to grown-ups: Remember this, if you are cradling me, it's about twelve inches between our faces . . . this is the distance I can see. So hold me as long as you want! I'm enjoying this.

Checklist of Hospital Essentials

Let's start at the top so to speak.

☐ Hairbrush

☐ Shampoo

☐ Hair clips/Hair bands (You may want to tie your hair back and make life as easy as possible.)

☐ Hair dryer

☐ Eye glasses/contact lenses/contact case/solution

☐ Soap

☐ Toothbrush

☐ Toothpaste

☐ Deodorant

☐ Body cream

☐ Lip balm (After hours of eating ice chips, you'll need this.)

☐ Comfy shirt you will want to wear during labor

☐ Pajamas (They should button in front.)

☐ 2nd pair of pajamas (If we need to stay an extra day or two in the hospital, you'll be happy about this one.)

☐ Bathrobe

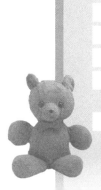

Nursing bra (Let's make things easy right from the start.)

Breast pads

Shirt (People will be coming to visit and you may want to change out of your pajamas for a few hours.)

Underwear

Loose pants (Again, I may have visitors and you may not want to wear pajamas for the next 2-4 days.)

Slippers (For visiting me in the nursery.)

Flip-flops for taking a shower

Socks (If it's winter, you'll want these.)

Going-home outfit (Pick something comfortable.)

Hospital pre-registration form (Fill out anything you can ahead of time.)

Insurance card

Essentials for Daddy

PJ's (Is he staying overnight at the hospital? Let's take care of him, too.)

Robe

Extra outfit. He may not have time to run home; he needs to make sure he packs a change of clothes.

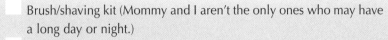

Brush/shaving kit (Mommy and I aren't the only ones who may have a long day or night.)

Slippers (Why can't Daddy be comfy, too?)

Watch with a second hand. (To time contractions.)

Favorite snacks (Daddy may not want hospital food.)

Luxury Items

Tape/CD player (If the hospital doesn't have this, you may want this during labor.)

Tapes/CD's (Even if the hospital has a player, you are going to want your own choice in music.)

Baby journal (Why not start recording my life right from the beginning?)

Playing cards/book/games (If you have a long labor, you'll want something to take your mind off of your pain. You and Daddy may have several hours to sit and wait for my arrival. Have some fun.)

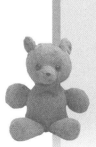

Important Items

☐ Car seat

☐ Camera (You're so busy, I don't want you to forget to capture the moment.)

☐ Video camera (Why not make me a star?)

☐ Film (What's the point of the camera if you don't have enough film?)

☐ Video cassettes (You may be recording for longer than you think.)

☐ Charger and video battery (It won't charge by itself.)

☐ Address book (You'll want to call everyone you know to tell them about my arrival—prepare a list of people you must call from the hospital. You're bound to forget someone if you aren't prepared ahead of time.)

☐ Phone card (How are you going to pay for all of those phone calls?)

☐ Empty duffel bag/suitcase (The hospital will provide you with some goodies to take home and friends may be bringing me some gifts. How are you going to manage to get everything out of the hospital?)

☐ A box of candy for the nurses who take care of me

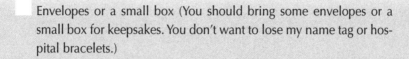

Envelopes or a small box (You should bring some envelopes or a small box for keepsakes. You don't want to lose my name tag or hospital bracelets.)

Essentials for Me

Baby bunting or outfit (My special outfit for coming home for the first time. This should be saved forever.)

Undershirt

Sweater

Socks/booties (Heat escapes through my extremities.)

Hat

Blanket (You will want to keep me warm and cozy.)

Don't Forget the Following at the Hospital

"It's a boy/girl card"

Hospital bracelets

My hospital hat

My hospital undershirt

Write down the names of the nurses for my baby book

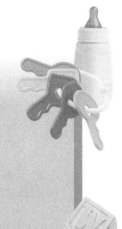

☐ Diapers from the cart in the room
☐ Wipes from the cart in the room
☐ Ointment from the cart in the room
☐ Changing pads (Again, these are in the cart in the room.)
☐ Extra formula if you are supplementing
☐ Fill out the birth certificate

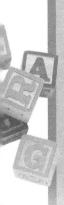

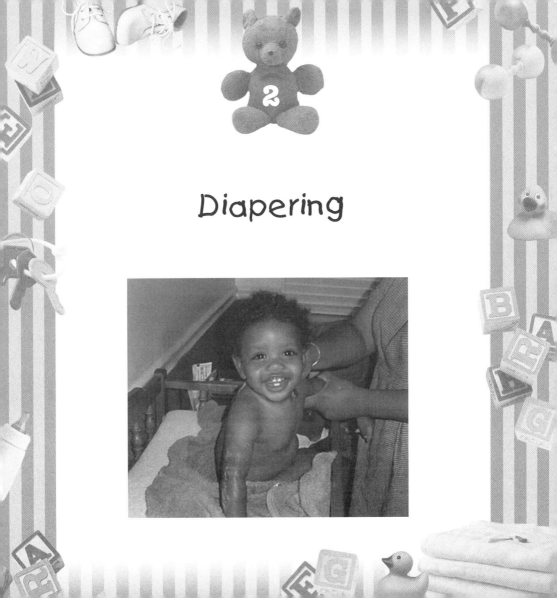

2

Diapering

When it comes to diapers, you have a choice to make—cloth diapers or disposable? If you choose cloth diapers, you can save money and be kind to the environment. You can hire a service or clean these yourself. Disposable diapers are more expensive but they go in the garbage and not the laundry. There is a positive side to each of them. You have to decide which one you feel is good for you—or rather, me!

Let's start with the basics. If you are using disposable diapers, remember that the tape goes in the back and the pattern goes in the front. (Could they make it any easier?)

Why do you always act so surprised when I have an accident? You know when the cold air hits it's bound to happen. Try strategically placing an extra diaper over me while you're changing me. Not only

21

will it keep me warm and perhaps prevent an accident, it can protect you in case I spring a leak.

Ouch . . . that hurts! Don't let that diaper tape stick to my skin. When the tape starts sticking to my skin, it means that it's time to buy bigger-sized diapers.

If you are using cloth diapers don't forget to buy diaper covers. How do you think you stop them from leaking? They actually make cloth diapers with covers attached to them. If you're worried about my little messes, you can even buy flushable liners for cloth diapers.

Here's a tip for Dad: My diaper rash cream doubles as a great aftershave lotion. I won't tell anyone if you won't.

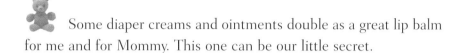

Some diaper creams and ointments double as a great lip balm for me and for Mommy. This one can be our little secret.

Did you know that there are two kinds of diaper rash? I guess that's bad news for me. It may be worse for you, as I may not be the bundle of joy you're used to seeing every day.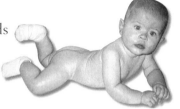

One kind of diaper rash is known as a chemical rash. This occurs when the acid contents in my stomach come out to form a rash on my skin. This rash is red and looks like a mild burn, and let me tell you, it hurts!

If I have a chemical rash you may want to try something called Triple Paste. Sometimes you can only find it behind the pharmacy counter so you may have to ask your pharmacist. Sometimes this cream needs to be ordered, so it's best to have some on hand in case

of emergencies rather than waiting for the emergency to occur. Prevention is worth an ounce of diaper rash cream.

The other kind of rash is a yeast diaper rash. This is when yeast overgrowth creates a red speckled rash that looks like red raised dots. There is a chance I may get this type of rash because yeast grows in a warm moist area, so until I'm pottytrained, we are fighting a losing battle. The yeast rash is best treated by an anti-fungal cream.

Open up the new diaper and have it ready before you change me. Better safe than sorry!

I know it's convenient to have baby oils and powders on the changing table. Did you know some of these items can be harmful to me if I swallow them? Don't tempt fate—keep these things out of my reach because they look like fun and interesting toys to me.

Note to grown-ups: Cornstarch can be very harmful if ingested, as well as baby oil. Keep them out of my reach.

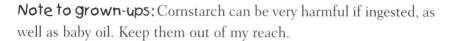 Trying to change a baby can be like wrestling a kangaroo on caffeine. If you don't want me to squirm, distract me by hanging a toy over the changing table, or at least hand me a toy. I hate staring at the ceiling.

If something is hanging above the changing table, make sure it's not low enough for me to get tangled. Even though you are right next to me, I can easily get caught in a curtain cord or a pull string.

Note to grown-ups: Don't put shelves above the changing table. If something falls it's landing on me, not you.

If I'm younger than two months please make sure the mobile isn't hanging directly over my head. Place it to my left or right side. For some reason I will cry if it's placed over the middle of my head.

It's neurological overload of some kind. I don't know why and the experts aren't quite sure either.

There's a safety belt on the changing table and my squirming is driving you nuts. Coincidence? I wonder. Why not make life easier and safer at the same time? Strap me on in.

As I get older, I'll squirm even more, so you should really try to make this seem like the best time in the world before I'm old enough to know better. Make it fun by singing a song or distracting me with a toy.

Always have plastic bags in your diaper bag to use to throw away dirty diapers. You won't want to go into anyone's home or office and leave a smelly diaper. Just stick them in a small sandwich bag (or a larger one when I get older) and everyone will be happy. I want to leave a good impression (and nothing else)!

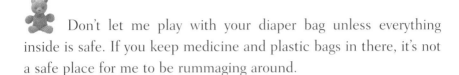

Don't let me play with your diaper bag unless everything inside is safe. If you keep medicine and plastic bags in there, it's not a safe place for me to be rummaging around.

Always make sure you have four or five diapers in your diaper bag—you really can never have too many. I may seem like a one- or two-diaper baby, but as I start eating strange foods and getting older you'll be surprised by the results of my digestive system.

Restock my diaper bag every night. You don't want to be in the middle of changing me, reach for a wipe and find none left.

Keep fever-reducing medicine, a decongestant and teething medicine in your diaper bag. You never know when you're going to need it. Always be ready for every emergency. Buy a diaper bag with plastic lining rather than cloth. You'll find out why.

As I get older, I'll get even more fidgety during changing time. If you are worried about me falling off the changing table, or if you just want to make your life a little easier, try changing me on the floor. It won't be great on your back but it's easier than trying to calm me. If I fidget while I'm on the floor, no one gets hurt . . . least of all me. Make sure you have a mat of some kind under my tushie.

No matter what else is going on around you, don't ever take your eyes off me—not for one second!

Surprise me! Have toys in the diaper bag that you can give to me when we're on the move and you're changing my diaper. You can rotate my toys so you aren't always giving me the same one or you can surprise me with my very favorite. You will need a bag full of tricks, so to speak. It's hard to be out in public during a squirmy diaper change. Believe me, the new environment will have me moving around even more than usual.

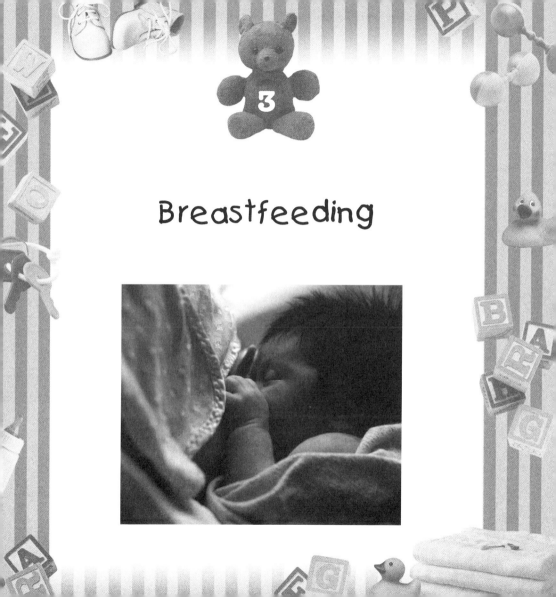

Breastfeeding

I'm glad you're going to breastfeed me because of the many immunities you're passing on. While commercials and movies may make it look like a piece of cake, sometimes it's not, so don't get discouraged. We have a long time to get it right and it's the best thing for me.

For the first three or four days, I won't be drinking breast milk. I'll be drinking something called colostrum that looks yellow and slightly thick. Breast milk doesn't come in for a few days. I don't think you'll have any trouble realizing its arrival. I've heard it's hard to miss.

Note to grown-ups: Colostrum is invaluable to me. Even if Mommy is having trouble breastfeeding, you can't replace the value of providing me with colostrum.

We may be home from the hospital before your milk comes in. It's important to have a support system already in place in case you have problems. Have the phone numbers of lactation specialists handy or supportive girlfriends who have been there. It's nice just to hear someone say, "Hang in there."

If you want to breastfeed me, keep at it in the beginning until your milk supply is full. If you give me an artificial nipple that's easier to latch onto, I may actually stop sucking and wait for you to give me a bottle . . . I may have been born yesterday, but I'm smarter than you think.

I know your back must be sore. Why don't you try bringing me to your breast rather than leaning over so much? I don't want an injured Mommy.

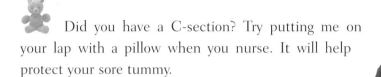

Did you have a C-section? Try putting me on your lap with a pillow when you nurse. It will help protect your sore tummy.

Did you know that improper latch-on is the main cause of nipple soreness? To prevent this, be sure to give me your nipple and as much of the area around the nipple as possible. But I don't need the whole thing—that would be an impossible feat.

I've heard it's a good idea to alternate breasts during each feeding or at every other feeding because you can become engorged. Don't forget to burp me . . . It's a good idea to do this each time you switch breasts.

Note to grown-ups: Most breastfed babies don't burp as much as formula-fed babies because we don't swallow as much air.

I know this takes some getting used to but it's no walk in the park for me either. It's going to take some time for me to figure out how to latch on correctly and how to suck and it's going to take some getting used to for both of us. I've been trying to tell you I'm hungry for twenty minutes, but you thought I was crying because I had a wet diaper.

 Did you know you can buy cream to help cure drying and chafing nipples? I know you're tired but you need to take care of yourself. I'm too young to take care of you and you need to stay healthy for the both of us. The best thing for sore nipples is pure lanolin, especially made for breastfeeding moms. Don't run out and buy any lanolin—it must be made for breastfeeding.

 Don't wait too long between nursing or pumping times because you can cause your milk supply to dwindle if you don't express your milk regularly—us babies usually need to eat every two to three hours in the beginning. Think of it this way: Breastfeeding is a matter of supply and demand—the more you nurse, the more you make.

When you're breastfeeding me, I love looking at your face (so there's where I got these good looks!). This is about as far as I can see for many weeks, so look at me, talk to me and smile!

Breastfeeding moms often worry that their babies aren't getting enough milk. But did you know that only one percent of women can't make enough milk? When I'm a newborn the best sign that I'm getting enough milk is that I have five to six wet diapers in a twenty-four-hour period. By the time I'm a week old, I should have six to eight wet diapers a day and two to three bowel movements. If I'm not having these, we both need to get some help.

To keep your milk supply up, you will have to pump every three hours. If you put pumped milk into bottles, Dad can feed me, too, and you can take a break. I'd like to start bonding with everybody in our family—and Daddy is so handsome!

You shouldn't wait until I'm crying to feed me. You don't wait for Daddy to cry to give him dinner, do you? As a general rule, for the first few months I'll be trying to eat every two to three hours.

Another reason you shouldn't wait too long between nursing times is because I will be hungrier and nurse even harder. If you don't want sore breasts, nurse more often, but for shorter lengths of time. Don't you eat faster when you're hungrier?

Note to grown-ups: Don't limit my sucking time. Us newborns may eat ten to twelve times in a twenty-four-hour period. Even if I suck a few minutes and fall asleep, I may wake up twenty minutes later and want to suck again. Don't fight it. You can try to nurse me every three hours during the night. We will probably begin developing a routine when your milk comes in. I know you need your sleep and I need mine, too.

To make your life as easy as possible, set up a nursing station or two nursing stations in our house. We're going to be spending a lot of time there, so why not have everything you need at your fingertips? Things like wipes, diapers, magazines or a book, water, TV or radio remote, juice, phone, change of clothes and burp cloths. You don't want to be jumping up and down looking for these basic items while trying to feed me. I know you are the queen of multitasking, but give yourself a break.

Don't feel guilty if you have a cup of coffee or glass of soda. You can eat or drink almost anything, but in small amounts. Hint: If you are worried about what you are eating or drinking, then have your coffee or wine *immediately* after you nurse me rather than before and in *moderation*.

Note to grown-ups: You have to watch your diet if I'm a highly allergic baby; otherwise, stop worrying so much.

I know mommies can't wait to fit into their pre-pregnancy jeans, but be sure to keep me well-nourished. Remember that mommies still need to eat more than they did before they were pregnant because they are still eating for two. The good news is, breast-feeding will help my mommy return to her normal weight faster. The better news is, Mommy will lose weight faster in those hard-to-lose places, like buns and thighs.

Let me throw you for a loop: I'm hungry . . . I'm hungry . . . I'm hungry. . . . Why am I nursing more often? I am probably having a growth spurt. This happens every so often and it has you thinking I'm not getting enough milk. Nope, I'm just growing.

Note to grown-ups: The first growth spurt usually occurs when I'm about two to three weeks old. During a growth spurt the supply temporarily isn't keeping up with the demand. If you nurse frequently for a few days the supply will meet the demand.

Here's a tip for you (you can thank me later). When your breast milk starts to leak (and it will—at the mall, at a party, in a meeting!) all you need to do is cross your arms or cross one arm and discreetly press down on your breast across the middle for two or three seconds and it will stop the leaking. Believe me, this is a tip you'll thank me for one day.

Want another tip that will make your life a lot easier? Wear something that pulls up from the bottom so nothing shows while you are breastfeeding. Some people think you unbutton from the top, but to be discreet it's easier to wear something you can slip me into from the bottom. Makes sense, doesn't it?

I know you don't even want to *think* about going back to work, but you need to if you plan to breastfeed me exclusively. Once your milk supply is established (two to three weeks after I'm born), you can start pumping to freeze for when you go back to work. It's best to prepare now. Do you have any idea how emotional you are going to be your first few days away from me?

When freezing breast milk, write the date you stored it plus the foods you ate that day. That way, you can use the oldest milk first and know if anything you ate upset my tummy.

You can store milk in a freezer that has a separate door for up to three months. You can keep it in the refrigerator for up to eight days if it's kept between 32–39 degrees F, but you have to play it safe and know our fridge is working correctly. If you are afraid the milk is no longer good you can smell it. One whiff of milk that's no longer good and you'll know it. If you have any doubts . . . the garbage is over there.

Now that you are storing breast milk, you will want to heat the bottles you're giving me. Never use a microwave oven to heat my bottles. Microwaves could leave hot spots in the milk that would burn my little tongue. You can boil my bottles in a saucepan, but please

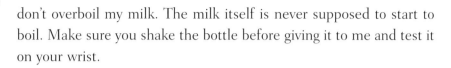

don't overboil my milk. The milk itself is never supposed to start to boil. Make sure you shake the bottle before giving it to me and test it on your wrist.

Remember, if you keep switching back and forth between a pumped bottle and breast before I am used to your breast, I may become confused. I don't ask you to drink from a cup one day and a bowl the next. Let me become comfortable with breastfeeding before giving me a bottle. This will work out much better for both of us.

Did you know if you rub my cheek a little when giving me the breast or the bottle it might get me to suck? If you try to have the same routine every time, I may feel more comfortable and understand when it's time to eat. Hint: In which direction do you want me to turn my head? Then rub this side of my cheek.

When I see Mommy, I expect the "real" milk. When you first introduce me to the pumped bottle, let Daddy or Grandma feed me.

I might not be as willing to take a bottle from Mommy because she has the good stuff. Buy bottles with nipples that look the most realistic to make it easier on me if you are supplementing and switching back and forth between breast and bottle.

Okay, so now I'm a little fussy when you nurse me because nursing may be more difficult than drinking from a bottle. You probably don't remember, but this nursing thing is a lot of hard work. Try using slower-flowing nipples when you bottle-feed me your pumped milk, so I still have to work when I suck. Otherwise, I may just want the bottle because it's easier.

Here's a hint, Daddy. Run the nipple of the bottle under warm water. I wouldn't give you a freezing cold glass to drink from (unless it's a beer).

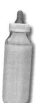

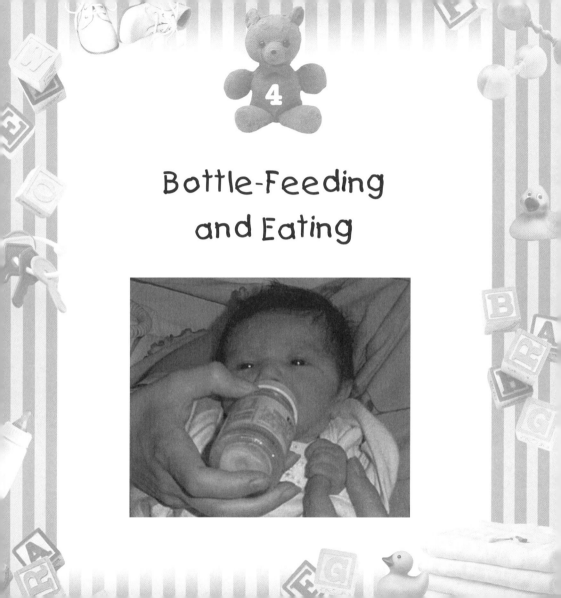

Bottle-Feeding and Eating

When I'm a brand-new baby I can only drink half an ounce and then I need to burp. Try burping me every half-ounce at first. As I get older I will be able to drink more before you have to burp me.

Do you know they make bottles that reduce gas by allowing less air in? Less air = less gas and we *both* like that equation. Don't buy the first bottle you see—we both deserve the best.

If we're using formula you need to follow the instructions provided on the can because some formulas need to be mixed with water and others don't. Check the expiration date on the can and wash the can before you open it. Now you can start preparing my meal.

When preparing formula with water, you should use cold water and let the tap run for two minutes. Old water pipes may contain lead and this will lessen the chance of lead contamination. No, I am not saying we have lead in our pipes; I am just saying to exercise caution. A little caution never hurt anyone . . . not that I know of anyway.

Formula does not necessarily need to be heated, but if you decide to do so, never use a microwave oven to heat my formula. If you boil my bottles, please don't make them too hot. You only need to heat my formula and you are only doing that because I may enjoy a warm meal. You can even simply run the bottle under hot tap water for a little while. If you are using powder mixed with water for my formula you need to determine the kind of water we have when preparing my formula. Some waters such as well water may need boiling.

Wait! Did you test that bottle before giving it to me? You need to shake out a few drops onto the inside of your wrist to make sure it's not too hot. It should be warm . . . not hot! Make sure you shake the bottle before giving it to me. Hey, I'm not asking you to prepare a seven-course dinner. This is a gourmet meal to me.

Now that you are supplementing breast milk with formula, I don't want to eat as often. Did you know that formula takes longer to digest than breast milk? I know because you keep trying to breastfeed me and I'm not hungry yet. If you think you're confused, imagine how I feel.

Don't roughhouse with me after I have a bottle. My food isn't digested and I'll spit up on you and me. I can't be responsible for the mess I make!

When I finish my bottle you can't save it for later; you need to throw the leftover milk away. You can never reheat or use unfinished formula. I'm not trying to be fussy, but no leftovers for me.

Look at the nipples and make sure they don't have any holes or tears that can break off in my mouth. If you think the nipple is getting old, you're right. Throw it away and get me a new one. I deserve the best.

Now that I'm five months old, you can stop taking that bottle out of my mouth to try to burp me. At this age I wait to burp until after I finish the whole bottle.

Hey, this nipple is for a three-month-old, and I am almost six months! Not only do you have to change the nipples for safety, you have to change them to keep up with me. There are different nipples for three months and six months, and so on, and I'm learning how to suck better every day. Throw away the old nipples every three months or so (or even more often to keep up with my ever-improving talents).

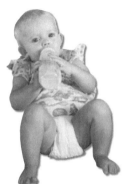

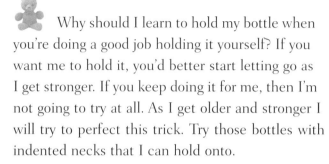 Why should I learn to hold my bottle when you're doing a good job holding it yourself? If you want me to hold it, you'd better start letting go as I get stronger. If you keep doing it for me, then I'm not going to try at all. As I get older and stronger I will try to perfect this trick. Try those bottles with indented necks that I can hold onto.

Note to grown-ups: Never, ever prop a bottle up for me to use. If I can't do it myself, you need to hold it for me because I can choke, as I have no way to remove the bottle from my mouth.

 In most cases, when I'm about six months old, our pediatrician will tell you that I'm ready for solid foods. I don't know why you call them "solid" foods; it just looks like mush to me.

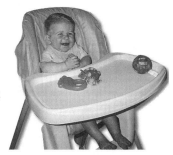

When I start eating solids, I'm not allowed to have any hard foods. When they say "solids," that's just a figure of speech; my food still needs to be very soft. Pretty confusing, huh?

My first "solid" or "not-so-solid" food will be rice cereal. Rice cereal is one of the least allergenic foods. If I am having trouble passing the rice you can switch me to oatmeal or barley. To help this little problem you can give me a little juice, such as apple or prune. Check with our doctor first as he will want you to wait until I'm at least four months old.

Am I ready for a high chair? If I can hold my head up and my tummy is strong enough, then I'm ready. Please remember that I have to be strong enough to sit up; otherwise I can fall out.

When I'm starting new foods you need to give me one food group at a time to make sure I'm not allergic. The doctor will guide you through this and tell you which foods and how long to do this, but I think you should feed me my veggies first. If you start me off on those yummy fruits then I'll never eat those veggies. If you're going to raise me to enjoy all kinds of foods, you're going to have to outsmart me—if you can!

I may not seem crazy about all the different foods you keep offering me. They make for great patterns on my clothes, though! Don't get frustrated when I'm not crazy about a particular food. You have your tastes, I have mine. Mine will change often, so if I refuse a food today, try me again next week.

Once I've tried each vegetable and fruit and you know I don't have any allergies, try mixing my favorite vegetable with one that I'm not so crazy about. If you always put my favorites together, then I won't like any of the new foods you give me. It's a good trick.

When I start eating fruits and vegetables, try not to give me the bottle first because then I won't be hungry. You can give me an ounce or two for the first few weeks to whet my appetite, but you really have to teach me that solid foods are my primary meal for the day.

When I'm done, I'm done. I might turn my head or close my mouth to let you know that I'm finished. Don't try to force-feed me because you might think I'm hungry. You have to be able to take a hint. If you try to force-feed me, then you'll be the one wearing my food instead of me for a change.

After I've mastered—and worn—fruits and veggies, the doctor will tell you when it's time for poultry and meats. No, I'm not going to be eating my way through a steak dinner. They make mashed versions of these foods, or you can find some instructions on how to

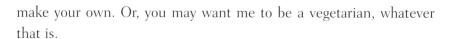

make your own. Or, you may want me to be a vegetarian, whatever that is.

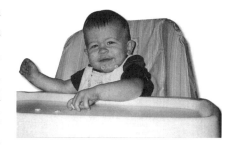

As I get older you can talk to the doctor about adding some things to my diet such as cheese and thin slices of turkey, but here's an example of some of the big no-no's for me: hot dogs, apples, popcorn, uncooked carrots, grapes, peanuts, raisins and chips. If you think a food is too hard for me, don't risk it. I have my whole life to try new foods.

Note to grown-ups: Don't give me whole slices at a time. I will definitely put too much food in my mouth, causing me to choke. Make sure I can handle the pieces you give to me.

How about some finger foods? I'm not talking about those little party sandwiches. At eight to ten months you can try giving me very small "O-shaped" cereal, tiny well-cooked pasta or some steamed soft vegetables. Again, check with the doctor to make sure I'm ready. By the way, the "O-shaped" cereal is a lot of fun for me and will be a big relief to you when I'm in one of those fussy moods.

Note to grown-ups: Eight months is generally fine to introduce me to cheese, cottage cheese and plain yogurt.

So, I'm not interested in eating today. Don't worry, I won't starve. Every baby is different and I may eat more for breakfast and less for dinner. Basically, if I refuse to eat lunch, I'll be begging (or rather crying) for food by dinnertime. It's important to try to maintain a schedule so you run the show rather than me. You can work with the doctor about when to start giving me more solids and adding a snack into my schedule.

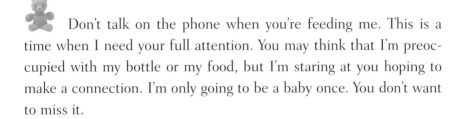

Don't talk on the phone when you're feeding me. This is a time when I need your full attention. You may think that I'm preoccupied with my bottle or my food, but I'm staring at you hoping to make a connection. I'm only going to be a baby once. You don't want to miss it.

Don't get mad at me for grabbing that spoon—it's so shiny. You want me to learn how to hold it, don't you?

It's not just the spoon I'm after. Of course I'm going to try to hold the bowl. I need to look in it to check out what you're feeding me. I want to see if it's really top quality. If you don't want a mess, then don't tempt me by putting that bowl right in front of my face. Babies = mess. If you didn't count on a mess, you're out of luck.

If you don't want me to be frustrated, try giving me a baby-friendly spoon made just for me. Baby spoons are slightly smaller and deeper than the ones grown-ups use. Don't ever feed me with plastic picnic spoons because they can crack and can be very dangerous. Always use a safe spoon I can't bite through.

Do you want to know why I cry when you wipe my face? I can't breathe! How would you like it if someone attacked your nose and mouth with a tissue? When you wipe my face, talk to me in a calm voice and tell me to "Breathe."

If we have a collapsible high chair or we're using a chair in a restaurant or friend's house, you need to make sure the chair is fully open and locked into place. Sometimes chairs look like they're open, when actually they're not. Please make sure my chair is fully locked into place. You don't want it to close when I'm sitting in it or see me folded in half.

Do you think it would be fun for me to use the food tray on my high chair as a diving board? I do! So always use the safety straps. You never know what I might be thinking.

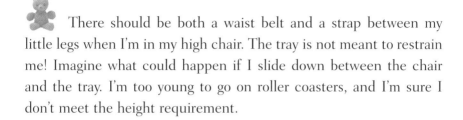

There should be both a waist belt and a strap between my little legs when I'm in my high chair. The tray is not meant to restrain me! Imagine what could happen if I slide down between the chair and the tray. I'm too young to go on roller coasters, and I'm sure I don't meet the height requirement.

Consider buying a high chair that has a wide base for stability and a post between my legs to prevent me from slipping. Yes, I know I'm strapped in, but a little extra safety never hurt anyone!

No one is allowed to lean or climb on my high chair. Don't let me play on it or try to climb into it myself. If these things are used improperly, they can tip over. Hey, it looks like a fun toy to me and you keep putting me in it, so why shouldn't I save you the time and do it myself?

When we're out in a restaurant, disposable bibs are great. You can even use them to clean my spoon when I finish eating. Then just throw the bib away and you don't have to put a messy bib in your diaper bag.

I'm strapped in my high chair correctly so you think it's safe to leave the room. Who are you kidding? I don't want to be stuck in here, especially if you're not around. It's never safe to leave me in one of these things by myself. Never put it by a table, counter or wall. I'll be able to push myself off and that's just asking for trouble.

As I get older, you might want to try plastic bibs rather than washing cloth bibs. The fabric ones are cute for when we're with company (I like it when you show me off!) but for convenience try a plastic bib.

I might want bananas for breakfast, but it's really up to you. Don't let me start controlling the menu. Otherwise, mealtime will become a nightmare. You control what I eat; I really don't know any better. Once you give me a choice, then I'll take over and you don't want that . . . do you?

Do not make mealtime into playtime. I will make such a mess and such a fuss. Mealtime is mealtime, and playtime is something totally different. Don't get me confused.

My dinnertime isn't always your dinnertime and I need to get used to that. I'll throw a tantrum while you're eating if you let me. If I've already eaten, then put me in a safe place while you have your dinner. Don't let me dictate your time. You set the rules (or at least I let you think you do).

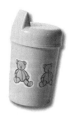

Be careful of relatives bearing nuts. (Although, from what I've seen so far some of our relatives may be nuts!) Some people have no idea that many foods are choking hazards to me. Always be sure to tell visitors that I'm not ready for grown-up food yet and tell them exactly what they can give to me. You'd be surprised how many people think they can appease me with food without even knowing what I can eat.

At about six months the doctor will tell you to have my sippy cup ready during mealtimes. You should try a two-handled spillproof cup to start. Since I've been drinking from your breast or a bottle, this will make the transition easier for me.

Note to grown-ups: Don't be discouraged if I don't master my sippy cup at first. I may not learn how to use it until I'm twelve months old or even eighteen months old. Remember, every baby develops differently. This doesn't mean I won't get into college.

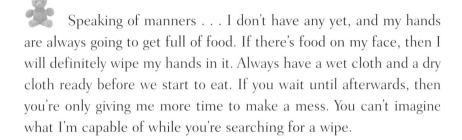

Speaking of manners . . . I don't have any yet, and my hands are always going to get full of food. If there's food on my face, then I will definitely wipe my hands in it. Always have a wet cloth and a dry cloth ready before we start to eat. If you wait until afterwards, then you're only giving me more time to make a mess. You can't imagine what I'm capable of while you're searching for a wipe.

Don't forget to brush my teeth after meals. Did you know they make toothbrushes for babies? You can start brushing them when I have about four to six teeth, but you can get me used to the idea even earlier by wiping my gums and beginning teeth gently with a wet cloth or gauze.

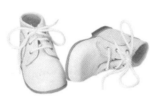

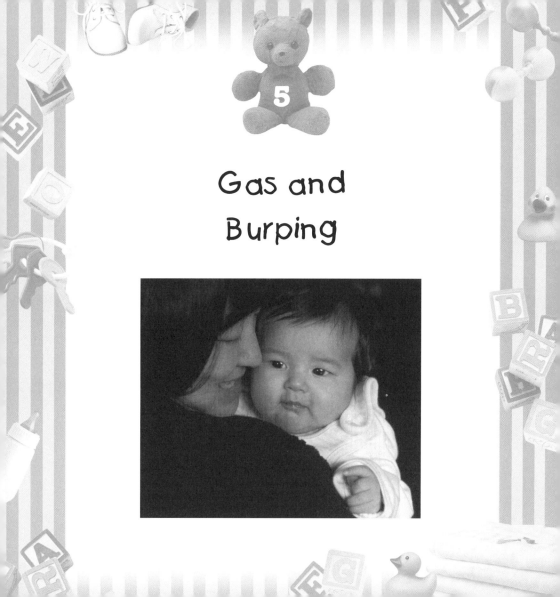

Gas and Burping

When feeding me, it's a good idea to try and burp me approximately every one to two ounces. You don't want to see how unhappy I'll be if you give me the entire bottle and then try to burp me. As I get older I'll be able to drink more before you burp me. Don't forget to burp me when I've finished the bottle as well.

Always have a burp cloth or towel handy. Would you rather wash your outfit or my burp cloth?

Hint: Friends and family may not remember to use a burp cloth, so give it to them . . . QUICK!

When you see me bend my legs a lot that probably means I'm gassy. Burping me will give me some relief.

Don't hit me so hard. How would you like it if I whacked your back after you ate? Gentle burping, please.

Sometimes when I'm crying you might rush to feed me, when what I actually need is to burp. If you feed me when I'm gassy it'll only make me feel worse.

Let me help you out: "Waaaah!" means I'm hungry. "Waaah!" means I'm gassy. See the difference?

I may cry when I'm hungry and crying could cause me to swallow air. Now that I've eaten and I'm well fed you need to know that the extra air I swallowed may cause some discomfort if we don't spend some time in one of the many burping positions.

Try rubbing my back; it helps me burp and it feels nice and cuddly, too. I might even fall asleep!

Of course I'm going to spit up the moment you remove the burp cloth. What's your rush? You should burp me for at least five minutes—and be prepared for me to spit up again another twenty minutes after that.

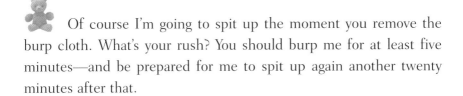

After burping me it's a good idea to keep me sitting upright for another fifteen minutes to avoid me spitting up. It's up to you . . . I'm not the one doing any of the cleaning up around here.

In addition to burping me over your shoulder, try other positions like holding me over your knee with my face down. It may seem awkward to you, but the pediatrician can show you how to do it. If nothing else is working, it may give me some relief . . . plus I get to check out what's on the floor.

When you're tired in the middle of the night, the last thing you probably want to do is burp me. Please take a little extra time to do this, even if I fall asleep. If you don't give me some relief now, we'll both pay later.

You're going to be tired during those late-night feedings but you need to stay awake to feed and burp me. After you feed me, don't be tempted to let me sleep in your bed! No matter how tired you are, you must return me to my crib or bassinet! If it's Mommy's turn to feed me and she's tired, she needs to ask Daddy for help and the same goes with you, Daddy!

If I have what's called gastric reflux—aka "spitting up like crazy"—you are definitely going to have to spend some extra time burping me to make sure the food doesn't come right back up. I know you're tired but you may have to spend thirty minutes or longer making sure that I'm okay.

Hopefully, I'll outgrow this soon. Most babies do. If it doesn't improve, you have any worries or I have "projectile vomiting" (you'll know if you see it!), call my doctor.

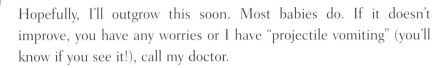 Everyone seems to think that if I cry I must be hungry or need a diaper change. Sometimes I just need a gentle burp. It's hard to get those things out on my own. Even if I'm not gassy, I might just like a back rub anyway. Don't you like a massage now and again?

Visitors love giving me a bottle, but they don't always like to burp me. You have to make sure that no matter who feeds me, some-one burps me. Otherwise, I'll feel like I'm going to explode . . . and I might just do that!

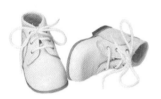

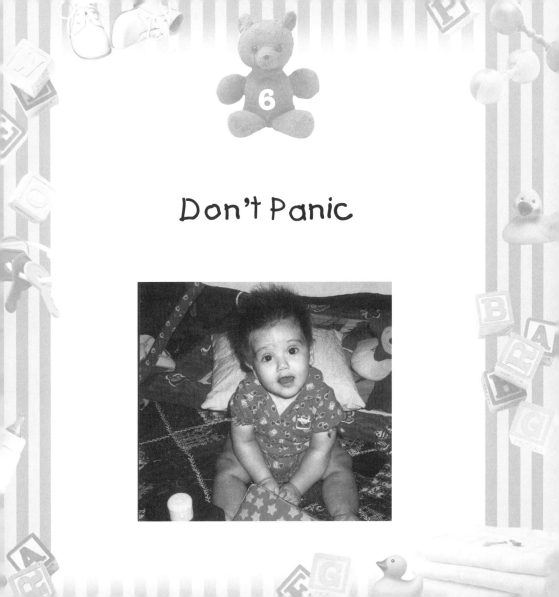

6

Don't Panic

Babies cry. That's what we do. Ever hear the saying "Don't cry like a baby"? So when I'm crying don't freak out. It's normal. I am just doing what I am supposed to do. You've never read a story in the newspaper about a baby who spontaneously combusted from crying. The fact is, I cannot hurt myself from crying.

Don't panic if I have a temperature. I am going to get sick. But if I have a fever, I'm fussy, can't sleep or if I'm too tired (confusing huh?), call the doctor. The doctor will tell you when my symptoms are cause for concern. Panicking doesn't help me. I'll recognize that look on your face and then we're both done for.

Note to grown-ups: You should always call the doctor if I have a fever or you are simply worried about me. Play it safe!

If you have an emergency, make sure you know how to save me. Learn CPR (cardiopulmonary resuscitation) for infants—it can be a lifesaver when seconds count.

Note to grown-ups: Taking a short class at our local hospital could save a life.

Oh no, what is that flaky stuff on my shoulders and head? Take me to the hairdresser . . . quick! Actually, I'm just kidding you. What I have is called cradle cap, which is an irritation of my scalp like dandruff. It's usually not itchy and it doesn't hurt me at all. Simply continue to use regular baby shampoo and gently wash my head with a soft washcloth.

You locked me in a running car? (Okay, panic a little bit but remain calm!) If it happens you can rescue me quickly if you give an extra set of keys to a few different friends and family

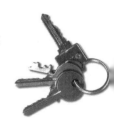

members and hide a key in the house. After reading this book you'll know I should never be left alone in the car, whether it's running or not.

If you walk outside to get the mail and the door accidentally closes behind you—also panic! Hopefully, you decided to get the mail while I am safe in my crib during naptime and you have the baby monitor in your hand as you're walking to our neighbor's house to get our spare key. Right?

Note to grown-ups: Play it safe. If you're going outside, even for a moment, take me with you. The same applies if we're playing outside and you need to run in the house to get something. Where you go, I go!

Please don't compare me to other babies. I don't compare you to other parents! If I don't have a tooth before my first birthday, it doesn't mean I will grow up with no teeth! If I'm not speaking French by the time I'm one, please don't take me to a speech pathologist! If I haven't read *War and Peace* by the time I'm six months old, it doesn't mean I'm not a genius . . . so don't panic!

So you need to get showered for work and I'm crying? Put me in my car seat and bring me in the bathroom. Sometimes the sound of the water soothes me right to sleep. Just be careful where you place me so that I am not holding anything dangerous. Make sure you can see me at all times.

Don't panic if you hear these words from my pediatrician: "Your baby has colic." Colic is the word the doctors use to explain why I'm crying at the top of my lungs day and night, depriving you of your crucial beauty sleep. Some doctors say colic is caused by the underdevelopment of my digestive system and others attribute my constant crying to gas. The good news is that it should only last for about three months . . . the bad news is that it can last for about three months. In any event, you won't be getting much of that beauty sleep, so try to avoid mirrors for a while.

Note to grown-ups: Hold me tummy to tummy and walk with me. I like this warmth. Even though the colic is still causing me pain, I will learn that you care that I'm hurting. Don't be surprised if the colic lasts more than three months. It lasts longer in some babies.

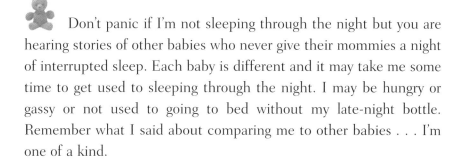

Don't panic if I'm not sleeping through the night but you are hearing stories of other babies who never give their mommies a night of interrupted sleep. Each baby is different and it may take me some time to get used to sleeping through the night. I may be hungry or gassy or not used to going to bed without my late-night bottle. Remember what I said about comparing me to other babies . . . I'm one of a kind.

Don't panic if you need to take me on an airplane—even if our seatmates seem less than thrilled as we sit down. Have a bottle ready for me to suck on during takeoff and landing to help my ears. Be sure to wait until we're actually taking off or I may finish it too soon.

Note to grown-ups: If you ask the flight attendant to warm my bottle, please make sure it isn't too hot.

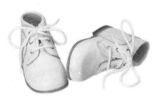

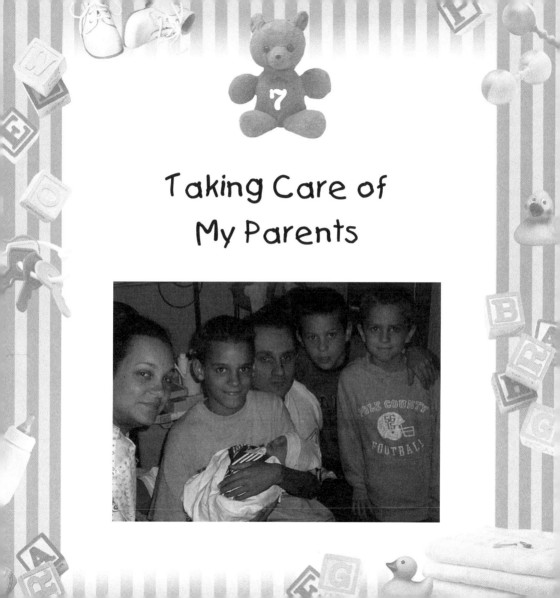

Taking Care of
My Parents

For all of the daddies . . . take care of Mommy; she's exhausted!

A foot massage is needed during pregnancy and after pregnancy as well. Mommy's feet keep changing shape and size.

Mommies need to rest during the first couple of days after giving birth to me. The truth is, mommies won't get a full night's sleep for at least six months and generally sleep with one eye open until their babies go to college.

In the first few months of my life, I will wake up every three to four hours for a bottle (or even more). Some people think they should eat when I eat. I have a better idea: You should sleep when I sleep. Take catnaps whenever I fall asleep because you need to be alert when I'm awake.

 Here's a tip for the visiting relatives—give the mommies or daddies some time alone. This is their special time. It's not the time for them to be making coffee and serving ladyfingers.

Try alternating feeding shifts between Mommy and Daddy. Mommy gets the midnight and 7 A.M. feedings and Daddy can feed me at 4 A.M. or vice versa. If you do three shifts in a row, you won't be any good to me or anyone else.

Note to Mom: Good luck getting Daddy to move at 4 A.M.

Mommy, are you feeling a little strange? I bet you're thinking you should be feeling at ease now that I've entered the world. That's not always the case. You have something raging through you called hormones. These can cause mood swings and postpartum depression. If you are worried about how you are feeling, or you absolutely can't

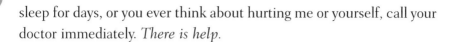

sleep for days, or you ever think about hurting me or yourself, call your doctor immediately. *There is help.*

Even if your hormones aren't affecting you, you might feel like you're having an identity crisis. You've gone from driving a sporty car to a minivan and you've traded your designer bag for a diaper bag. It will take a while for you to adjust to "mommyhood," but you will—and you'll be great. Remember to thank me for it.

Mommy, I've heard you complain to Daddy that you're discouraged because you can't fit into your pre-pregnancy jeans and you feel fat. (I'll have to remind him he needs to be quicker in his reply!) It took time to gain the weight and it will take time to take it off. If you're going to take care of me, you need to stay healthy and not try any of those ridiculous crash diets.

Hint: Don't eat when I eat because you'll be eating all day.

Mom, I know you are feeling a little lost at times . . . it's only natural. Unfortunately, I don't come with an instruction booklet. Use your natural instincts. Don't worry. I won't break.

 Daddy may be feeling left out or a little lost as well. He and I naturally don't spend as much time together. Daddy needs to have his own little jobs when it comes to taking care of me. For example, he can be in charge of bath and bedtime. I'd love to have Daddy read to me.

 Have the in-laws become outlaws? Sometimes we count on family members to help but it's a little more than we bargained for. We are spending our first few moments as a family together and you may not always want a constant flow of people in the house. Everyone will understand your feelings as long as you explain that we'd like some time to bond. Don't keep it bottled in. . . . That must hurt!

 Mommies and Daddies need to work together as a team. You

are going to see Daddy doing things that make you want to scream and he will see you doing things that make him want to scream. Remember—you both have one mission—taking care of me!

I know I'm cute but don't get suckered into those phone calls by portrait studios saying that we have been selected for a free portrait at your home. Once you see those cute test shots of me you won't be able to resist and $900 later you will have the same thing you could have gotten somewhere else for $9.99.

Get a baby-sitter! Believe me, I will survive a few hours without you. Mommies and daddies need some time alone together. You know Grandma and Grandpa have some child-care experience of their own, so give them a ring and go out for a nice dinner. If you feel guilty about leaving, trust me, I'll give you a list of things to feel guilty about when I become a teenager. So, for now, take advantage of the fact that I don't talk yet.

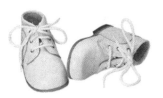

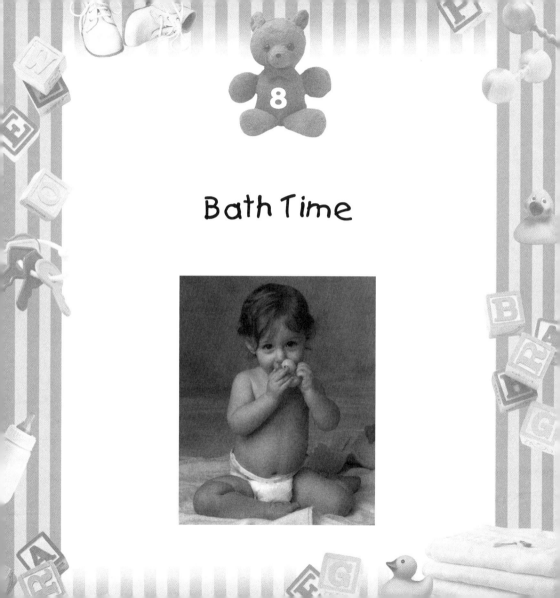

8

Bath Time

NEVER take your eyes off me when I'm in the water. Not unless you see the Tooth Fairy, the Easter Bunny, Santa Claus, Peter Pan and Mother Goose all on the same day . . . and not on or including October 31! Use a lot of caution and always hold me with at least one hand.

Always check the temperature of the bath water with your wrist before putting me in. If you still aren't sure, try your elbow. The water may seem okay when you are filling the tub, but as you know from hot water surges in the shower, anything can happen. See page 193 for information on burn prevention.

I love bath time, but you might not love getting soaked, too. Don't wear your nice clothes while you're giving me a bath.

Have everything ready and waiting from a towel and shampoo to washcloths. Everything should be at your fingertips. Don't make yourself reach for anything. I repeat: "Never turn your back on me."

Don't take my diaper off until we get to the bathroom. Do you really want to clean up a mess? I know you always think I can hold it but you're really expecting too much out of little old me.

When I get older and I can sit up on my own, give me some toys to play with. It makes bath time more fun for me and I can explore something new at the same time.

If you use a baby bath seat, be aware it is *not* a safety device—it is meant to give you a hand with a squirmy baby (is that me?). Baby bath seats come with some hazards you need to be aware of at all times. Bath seats can tip over; my little legs can slip through the leg holes; and when I'm older, I may try to climb over the seat and fall into the tub.

A note to grown-ups: The CPSC is in the process of setting a federal safety standard to make baby bath seats safe.

Never leave me alone in the tub. Always keep me within arms' reach. Even though I'm slippery when wet, I'm not a fish and I don't know how to swim. I can't even drink water out of a glass yet!

So, the phone is ringing. What's more important than keeping your eye on me in the bathtub? They'll call back. And if the person at the door is really important, they'll wait. Nothing is more important than staying with me when I take a bath. If you leave, I will try to follow.

Never leave me alone with a sibling. He/she can barely lift him/herself out of the bath. How do you expect my brother or sister to lift me out if there's a problem?

If you've decided to use a bath seat to help hold me while you bathe me, take every precaution. You know those suction cups at the bottom of my bath seat? They need to be attached to the smooth surface of the tub. Just because my seat has suction cups, it doesn't mean they will stay in place on any surface. Unfortunately, if the tub is a nonskid or slip-resistant tub, my seat will skid and will slip. I know it's a little confusing. A bath seat can become dislodged and it should *never* take the place of adult supervision.

Here's a tip: Remember to clean these seats frequently.

Never give me a sponge to play with. I will put it in my mouth and break some pieces off. This is an even easier trick when the sponge is wet. Just stick with using a washcloth.

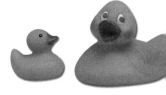

Make sure all bath toys are age-appropriate. It's difficult enough when I break off a small piece of a toy when I'm not in the tub. Can you imagine what a problem we're going to have if you give me a dangerous toy when I'm in the tub?

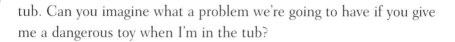 Bath soaps help me relax and put me to sleep. Try them too, Mommy, you look exhausted! You really should try to get a good night's sleep once in a while.

Here's a great tip from my mommy. When I outgrew my bassinet, my mommy took the mattress pad and put it on the floor next to the tub during bath time. With my bath towel over the mattress pad, I go from the tub to a soft towel with a cushion underneath.

When you take me out of the bath and I start crying, do you know what I'm saying? Let me translate: "I'm cold, I'm cold, I'm cold!" Have my clothes ready and waiting. Do you have any idea how cold I am with you holding me up in my birthday suit while the water drips everywhere? My hair's wet and for some weird reason my body won't stop shaking. What's that all about?

Make sure the bathroom rug won't slip and cause me (or you holding me) to fall. All you need is some tape or nonslip mats. Or make your life even easier and take the rugs out altogether until you can make sure they won't slip under our feet.

Yes, you need safety latches in the bathroom, too. I think that blue liquid I see you swallowing looks really good. I might like to try some when you are busy getting my bath ready.

Keep the national toll-free number to the Poison Control Center near the phone: 1-800-222-1222. You can call anytime from anywhere in the U.S., and they'll connect you to the nearest poison center.

Make sure you put safety latches on the toilet seat as well. It looks like an easy place to drop a toy. Now, how am I going to get a toy out of that thing? I guess I just have to reach for it. My head is heavier than the rest of my body and if I fall I'm going in headfirst.

Anytime is bath time as far as I'm concerned, but you might want to bathe me at night because I usually fall asleep afterwards. Baths are so relaxing.

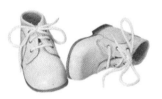

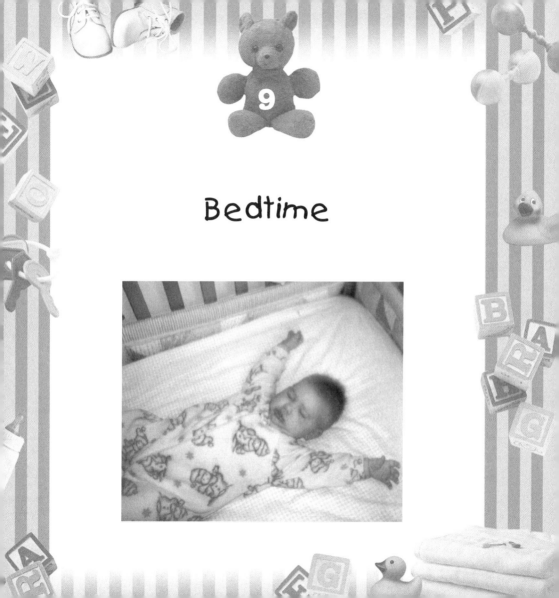

Bedtime

I really can be a low-maintenance newborn. Here's how: I really love my bassinet. It's small and I love sleeping in your room. A good trick for mommies and daddies is to rock my bassinet a bit when I'm fussy in the middle of the night. If you keep it close to your bed you don't even have to get up. Just rock me gently while you rest.

There are all sorts of rules as to how I should or shouldn't sleep. Remember to put me on my back on a firm, tight-fitting mattress so I can't slip into any cracks. Remove pillows, quilts, comforters and sheepskins from the bassinet or crib—so I don't get caught in them and suffocate.

Since the American Academy of Pediatrics recommended in 1992 that infants be placed to sleep on their backs, the SIDS (sudden infant death syndrome) rate has decreased by more than 40 percent. The AAP helped launch the Back to Sleep Campaign so you'll remember that at bedtime or nap time *the safest way for me to sleep is on my back.*

Don't leave stuffed animals or toys with plastic buttons, eyes or noses I can pull or choke on in the crib. That furry creature can cover my mouth and nose when I sleep and make it hard to breathe.

If you decided to buy a bassinet with all of those pretty bows and ribbons you have to make sure they are either cut short, fastened very tightly, or removed so I can't pull them off or become tangled in them.

Does my bassinet fold? If so, make sure it's locked firmly in place before you put me in it. That's not the only thing that needs to be locked. I think I feel my bassinet moving back and forth. That swinging feature needs to be locked before you put me to sleep.

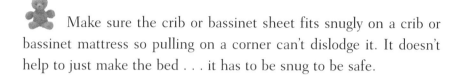

Make sure the crib or bassinet sheet fits snugly on a crib or bassinet mattress so pulling on a corner can't dislodge it. It doesn't help to just make the bed . . . it has to be snug to be safe.

If you don't have a clean baby sheet, an adult sheet is never an option. It can come loose and become dangerous for me. . . . You wouldn't sleep with a baby sheet, so don't expect me to use one of your oversized ones.

Never place the crib or bassinet next to window blinds or curtain cords. I can reach them when you aren't looking. Remember that everything looks like a fun toy to me. I shouldn't be able to reach my mobile either. It's fun to look at but no touching!

The spindles in the bassinet should be no farther apart than 2⅜ inches and the same goes for the slats in the crib. If you can fit a soda can through any of the slats, then the opening is too big.

Crib gyms need to be secured to the crib at both ends. I should never be able to pull this or any toy into my crib. Toys that stretch across the crib with string, cord or ribbons are hazardous to more active and older babies.

No strings with loops or openings and no cords should hang into the crib. I like to grab everything and there's no reason to give me such dangerous items to play with. My crib should be the safest place. You aren't there twenty-four hours a day to monitor me. You need to feel as safe leaving me there as I feel being there.

Note to grown-ups: A baby monitor is a great investment that will give you peace of mind in knowing you'll hear me when I need you.

When you are deciding which toys you want to put in my crib, you need to remember never to use toys with catch points that can hook my clothing. I don't know what I'm doing and if a toy has something that can get snared onto my clothing . . . I will get caught.

Us babies generally sleep through the night by about four to five months old . . . but that's generally. All babies are different and I like to think I broke the mold when I was born. To help me learn to sleep through the night, talk to the doctor about slowly increasing the amount of food I eat at my nighttime feedings. When the doctor says I'm ready, as you slowly increase the food, I will sleep a little longer with each increase. Again, remember all babies are different and there may be a good reason I am not sleeping through the night. Some babies don't sleep through the night until they are eight or even ten months old.

When I'm old enough to sleep in my crib we're going to play all sorts of games . . . control games, that is! I just want you to stay in the room or take me out of the crib and hold me. Once I'm six months old, don't give in to these games. I need to learn that bedtime is bedtime.

I know that old antique crib is cute and that you can save money by putting me in a used crib . . . but is it safe? There can be missing or broken pieces or damage to these cribs. You might not hear me crying for help in the middle of the night. Standards for cribs have changed since the 1970s and 1980s. Would you want to sleep in an unsafe bed?

Corner posts may look fancy but they can be dangerous. You will usually find these on older cribs. Here's where my math comes in handy. . . . If we have a crib with these posts, they should be less than $\frac{1}{16}$ of an inch high. Never put me in a crib that has decorative knobs on corner posts. If we have a crib with these knobs, they should be unscrewed or sawed off so they are flush with the head- and footboards.

Note: After sawing these off, you will need to sand the crib for splinters or sharp corners.

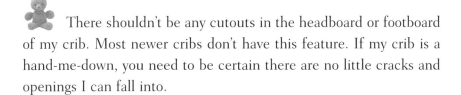

There shouldn't be any cutouts in the headboard or footboard of my crib. Most newer cribs don't have this feature. If my crib is a hand-me-down, you need to be certain there are no little cracks and openings I can fall into.

If my older crib was made before 1978, it may have been painted with something called a lead-based paint. I don't know what it is, but it doesn't sound good to me. You know how I like to put everything in my mouth. If the crib has lead-based paint then it's time to get a new crib.

Every once in a while you'll need to check the screws, nuts and bolts on my crib to make sure nothing is loose. Make sure the support system for my mattress is secure and that nothing is broken or bent that would allow my mattress to fall. I'm not asking you to walk around with a tool belt, but you do need to check these things often.

You need to constantly check the crib to make sure there are no rough edges, splinters, cracks in the wood or sharp points that could hurt me.

Try reading me a book before bedtime. If you teach me a routine and we stick to it, then I'll begin to know that bedtime is coming soon. If you just plop me in my crib, I can promise you one thing . . . I will cry. As I get older, I will try to alter any routine you set. Isn't that part of the game?

Do you sleep in your pants? Always put me in my pajamas. How would you like to sleep in the same clothes you've been wearing all day? PJ's are the most comfortable and they're safe to sleep in, too. Here's a tip: Put my PJ's on an hour before bedtime; don't wait for me to become cranky and difficult. Who knows, maybe I'll surprise you and fall asleep early for a change.

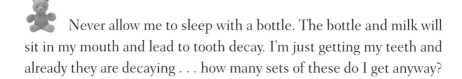 Never allow me to sleep with a bottle. The bottle and milk will sit in my mouth and lead to tooth decay. I'm just getting my teeth and already they are decaying . . . how many sets of these do I get anyway?

How about a little music? It'll help me fall asleep, and if you're on edge it'll calm your nerves as well. Plenty of toys play music; leave a couple in my room. Most toys these days even shut off automatically, so just flip the switch before you put me in bed. I'm a sharp cookie and I'll figure out how to turn them on without your help . . . eventually.

Don't leave me in the dark! If I can't see anything I'm going to be scared. A little night-light always helps. Sometimes I wake up in the middle of the night or early in the morning, and I have no idea where I am. I like to play by myself in the crib, but I can't enjoy this time (and neither can you) if I can't see anything.

Can you think of a better time for a back rub? Once I am able to roll over in my crib, start giving me short back rubs at night. Set the mood by turning on my night-light and then play some beautiful music. I love to hear you sing me a lullaby. I'll roll onto my tummy and get a great massage. It's so soothing. Maybe when I'm older I can do the same for you. . . .

I know it's fun to put me in your bed, but your bed has too many hidden hazards, such as soft bedding, pillows, thick quilts and comforters. Did you know that even the wall is dangerous? There is nothing stopping me from falling between the wall and the bed. . . . I fit into the tiniest spaces.

Okay, so you still want to cuddle me and I just told you that I should never be sleeping in your bed. I need to make this very clear . . . I should only sleep in a crib that meets current safety standards and has a firm, tight-fitting mattress. Your bed is a nice place to enjoy a bottle or a cuddle but let me sleep where it's safest. Don't you and Daddy need to start working on one of those sister or brother things?

At six months, just put me in my crib and walk out of the room when you put me down for a nap or bedtime. I'm old enough to try and trick you now and play some little games to get you back into the room. You have to let me know that it's bedtime and there's no fooling allowed.

Okay . . . so I still scream when you leave the room. If you pick me up every time I scream, I'll continue to scream. I don't know why I'm sleeping all by myself in this big prison with bars all around. Once I'm about five or six months old, you can try the Ferber Technique to get me to stop. For the first week or two, try coming back into my room every couple of minutes so at least I know you're still there. Wait five minutes and then leave; then come back ten minutes later.

You need to make sure that those latches that hold the crib sides up are sturdy and I can't open them and make a break for it. You do know NEVER to leave me in the crib with the side down . . . don't you?

When I'm five months old or when I'm able to push myself up on my hands and knees, you are going to have to take away my mobile and crib gym. I know I'm enjoying them but now they are no longer considered toys . . . they are considered hazards.

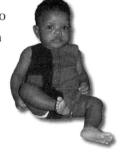

As soon as I learn to sit, you are going to have to lower the mattress so I can't fall out. By the time I learn to stand, the mattress needs to be at the lowest level. Don't wait for a potential accident before you lower the crib. You see how I'm learning to use my arms and legs. You need to stay one step ahead of me.

Do you know how to sneak out of a crib? Well, if you give me half a chance I'm going to learn how to escape. If you give me those bumpers that don't squish down, I'll show you how it's done. Crib bumpers MUST compress, otherwise I'll make a break for it. Do you have any idea how far it is from my crib to the floor of my room? It's farther than you think . . . especially for a baby. It may look close to you, but for me it's a few stories down. However, don't buy a very soft, flimsy bumper that could cover my mouth and cause me to suffocate.

As soon as I can stand up, you have to move the crib to the lowest position and remove the bumpers.

Here's a great tip: When I wake up in the morning, don't rush in to get me. I'm not always wide awake yet, and just like you, I might fall back to sleep. Unless I'm really grumbling or you feel I need your attention, just wait a couple of minutes. You might just get a few more winks yourself.

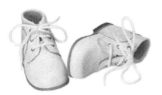

10

Getting Dressed
and Undressed

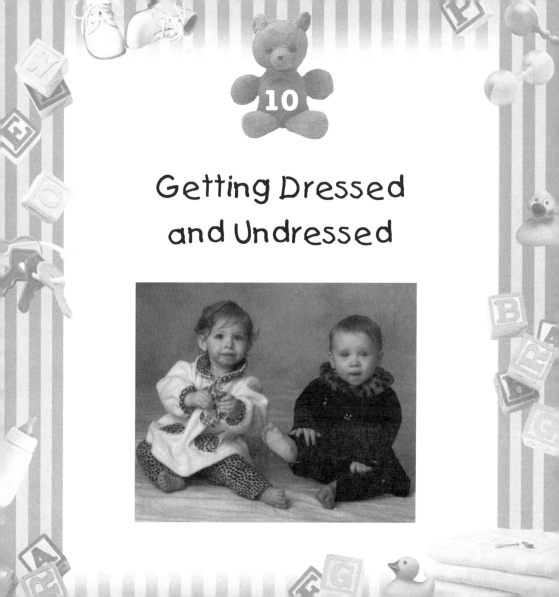

It takes some getting used to when it comes to dressing a newborn. Sometimes it's hard to learn how to put clothes on a little one, but I get dressed one leg at a time, just like you.

Once I get older I can help you if you help me. You need to teach me just how much fun getting dressed can be. Play peek-a-boo when you pull my shirt over my head. How would you feel if I was tugging at your clothes? Sometimes I get scared because I just don't know what you're doing to me. If you make changing time fun, I'll be more cooperative.

Some mommies like to dress girls with ribbons in their hair and in frilly dresses. Boys will have none of that, but one thing is the same for both girls and boys . . . we DON'T like socks.

So, here's a tip: Tuck our pants into our socks and they may just stay on longer. You have to make it as difficult as possible for me to pull those things off and put them in my mouth.

I do not like things on my feet! I've lost many shoes and I'm not even a year old yet. My mommy has a collection of single shoes and socks, if you think you may have a match. So, when you leave a store or someone's house, check to see that I have my booties and my hat. You wouldn't believe what I might leave behind.

Hats look adorable on me, I agree, but I hate wearing them! Don't get frustrated when I'd rather pull them off my head and use them as a teething ring. Here's a hint . . . take a picture! It'll last forever—unlike the hat.

Make sure if there is a little ball on top of my hat that it cannot come off. The same goes for buttons and any small items attached to clothes. If you feel anything is loose, either remove it so it's not a danger to me or exchange it for something without any dangerous attachments. Remember, anything near my mouth is making it in there. Anything I can pull off my clothes will also end up in my mouth.

Tell your friends and family not to buy any clothes with those tiny, tiny buttons. You don't have the patience for them, and neither do I. If your friends still buy them, maybe you should make them dress me!

Pick out my clothes *before* you bring me to the changing table. You won't have even one second to get something out of the closet. You can't turn your back on me, even for a moment. So, either pick my clothes out ahead of time or I'm coming with you on a field trip to the closet! How many times are you going to take me back and forth to the closet?

Take this advice: Really, I'm getting dizzy already.

If you plan on taking me someplace where you need me to behave, please dress me comfortably. I promise I won't be as cranky and everyone will compliment you on what a good baby I am. I know how you love to hear that! Besides, I've seen how cranky Daddy gets when he has to wear that thing around his neck that goes under his collar . . . he doesn't behave either when he has to wear that.

Overalls . . . these are a lesson in frustration. I know I look really cute in them, but don't even go there until you are better at dressing me. If you really must put me in this fashion statement, make sure you have the kind with the snaps at the bottom for easy access to my diaper.

Never put me alone in a playpen, a crib or anywhere with a bib or a necklace around my neck because these can get caught on all sorts of protrusions and cause me to choke.

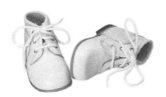

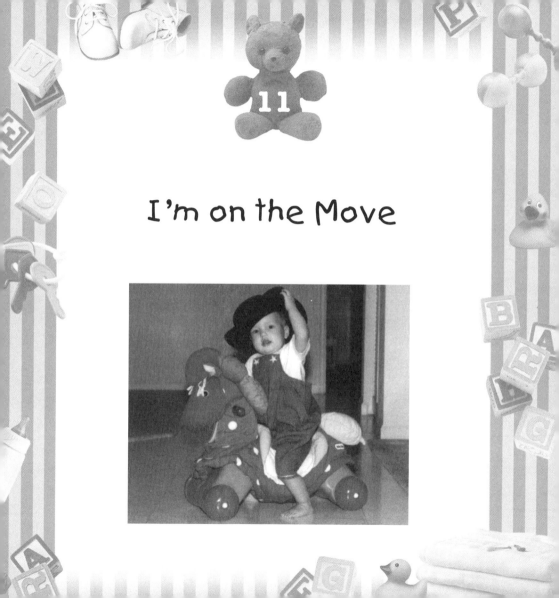

11

I'm on the Move

Once I begin to roll over, life as you know it is going to change . . . again. Keep an eye on me because sometimes I just can't stop rolling. I don't know where the "stop" button is.

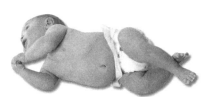

At three months I can really start moving my hands, and as time goes on, I will start reaching for everything. Never carry me and hot drinks or hot food at the same time. If you need some quick caffeine, you will have to decide: Carry me or the coffee mug, but never both!

Crawling is a wonderful thing! I get faster every day. It's a whole new world for me and I want to see it. I'm quite the explorer and I'll follow you into every room. It's time to baby-proof our home before I get into trouble. You can do this yourself or hire a professional baby-proofer.

 Don't leave anything on the floor that you don't want me to put in my mouth. Now that I can crawl, I'll look for anything new and interesting that I can suck on.

 Be wary of houseplants! When I see one of those pretty green things fall on the floor I want to grab it, play with it, and, of course—taste it. Either put those plants away from my play area, or get rid of the indoor kind and stick to the outdoor kind. I can swipe one of those leaves up off the floor without you ever noticing.

Note to grown-ups: You should learn which plants are poisonous and remove them from our home. See the list on page 192.

 First comes crawling; next comes standing. I'll try to pull myself up on anything. Please cover all sharp edges. Chances are I'll either hit my head on the way up or the way down.

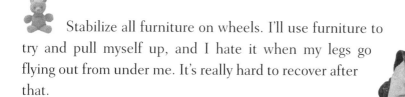

Stabilize all furniture on wheels. I'll use furniture to try and pull myself up, and I hate it when my legs go flying out from under me. It's really hard to recover after that.

Those baby walkers look safe don't they? Once I start moving, you better block off the stairs because you'll be surprised just how quickly I can find them . . . and walkers don't bounce . . . they crash. Use walkers only with adult supervision and very sparingly.

A walker is for flat surfaces only. You can be sure that I will find the one uneven part of our entire home. Keep me on flat surfaces and away from stairs, carpet edges and door thresholds.

Hopefully you didn't borrow my walker, since walker standards have changed since 1997. My walker shouldn't fit through a standard doorway or it must have "gripper strips" on the bottom to stop at the edge of a step.

When I travel in a walker you have to be even more aware of my surroundings. I can get to that hot oven door very quickly. I will try to get to anything that isn't pinned down, such as electric or drapery cords. If you leave the door open, I may even try to take a journey to the pool. Basically, you can't turn your back once I'm in my walker because I will try to explore everything and now I'm in a moving vehicle.

Instead of a walker, you may want to put me in a stationary activity center sometimes called a stationary exerciser. These are a lot of fun. I can bounce and play and I can't go anywhere. Basically, I'm stuck in this thing and you don't have to chase me around our home.

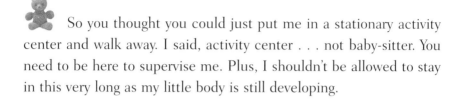

So you thought you could just put me in a stationary activity center and walk away. I said, activity center . . . not baby-sitter. You need to be here to supervise me. Plus, I shouldn't be allowed to stay in this very long as my little body is still developing.

I know you think if you put everything away in the cabinet, I won't find it . . . but you're wrong. As soon as I can crawl, I will open every door. Lock all cabinets containing cleaning products, knives, matches and plastic bags. They all look like fun toys to me. By now all of those cabinets are baby-proofed, right?

Never dispose of razor blades, toothbrushes and other dangerous items in bathroom or bedroom wastebaskets. Now that I'm crawling I will naturally look in the wastebasket, stick my hand in or tip it over. Be careful about what you throw in there. Throw all dangerous items in a wastebasket that I can't tip or reach into and make

sure it has a cover and is far, far away from me. If possible, put a wastebasket under the sink in a cabinet with a safety lock.

Keep me away from tablecloths so I can't pull hot food or liquids onto myself. Once I learn to pull, I will pull everything. A tablecloth looks like a blankie to me and I'm going to keep pulling on it until I get it.

Once I begin standing you need to fasten all furniture to the wall. This includes bookcases, TV stands, lamps and any shelving units or furniture stands. I may not be a good climber yet, but I am definitely a good tipper. I can tip almost anything over and it will fall right on top of me. So, if you want to keep your china and me in good shape, make sure I can't tip anything over.

Do we have a dog or cat? I know I have a stuffed version of those animals, but do we own the real thing? You need to keep the food bowl away from me as I may try to eat the dog food thinking if it's good enough for Rover, it's good enough for me. Hard dog food is a choking hazard. Also, check the floor frequently to see if Fluffy mistakenly bit off a piece of his dog cookie that's just waiting for me to sample—and choke on. Also, keep me away from the cat's litter box. I may try to play in that little sandbox. Why not? The cat seems to be spending a lot of time in there.

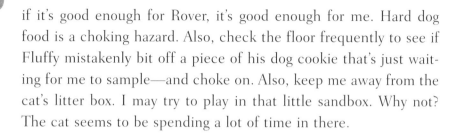

If we have pets they've probably developed an inferiority complex since I arrived on the scene. I sure hope they like being pulled because it's a lot of fun grabbing clumps of fur. I particularly like a game called chase the cat! Never leave me alone with a pet, and as I get older, teach me to "play nice."

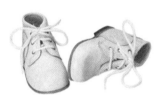

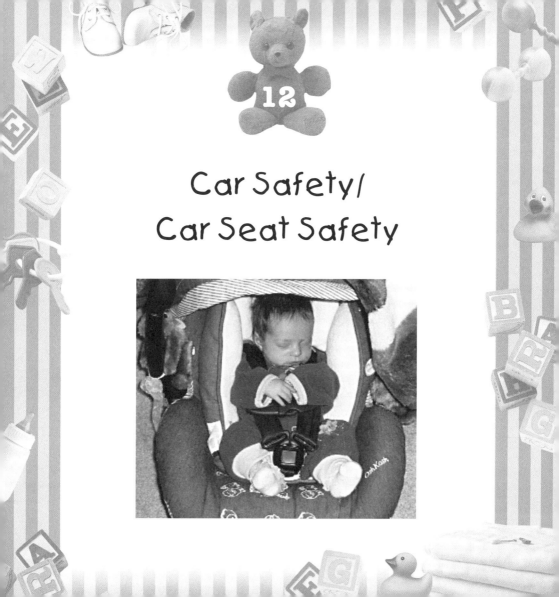

12

Car Safety/
Car Seat Safety

Here's a tough word for me: "instructions." I don't know what it means and apparently I take after Daddy because he hates them, too. All I know is that you must read these because they explain how to install and use the car seat. This isn't something you should guess at. You may think it's easy, but I don't want to become an experiment in trial and error. You remember how long it took Daddy to program the VCR *without* instructions, don't you?

Not to nag you, but did you install the car seat correctly? Eighty-five to ninety percent of all mommies and daddies get it wrong. You can go to college for a degree in car seat installation or you can call your local fire station or police department for help. I'll come with you. Those red trucks and those cars with the lights on top fascinate me. You can also find a certified technician in your neighborhood to inspect the installation of your car seat; go to *www.seatcheck.org* or call 1-866-SEAT-CHECK.

I see you and Daddy are high-fiving each other; but wait, you're not done yet. You need to read the seat belt and child seat–installation section in the owner's manual of your car. Not every car is the same and, unfortunately, the car seat can't install itself.

Remember, my car seat always goes in the backseat. It's the only safe place for me until I'm twelve years old. It's going to be a long twelve years. . . . I hope there's some entertainment for me back there.

We babies have made an amendment to the old saying, "Never look back." What it should say is "Always look back" . . . in the car, that is. I should never face forward in the backseat until I'm at least twenty pounds AND at least a year old. Don't feel bad; as far as I'm concerned you're the one who is facing the wrong direction.

If I weigh more than twenty pounds before my first birthday then you need to put me in a rear-facing convertible child safety seat. There are actually car seats for heavier (I prefer the term "physically advanced") babies. A convertible seat is one that can face the rear of the car but can turn to face the front of the car when I'm ready. Hey wow! My first convertible and I haven't even had my first birthday yet.

Note to grown-ups: Just a reminder, *I must be at least twenty pounds and a year old to face the front!*

When I'm riding in the car, please don't give me anything I can swallow. You can't reach me back here and if I accidentally swallow something, we're both in trouble.

My toys can become UFOs: Unusual Flying Objects. If you give me a toy, it must be a very soft plush toy.

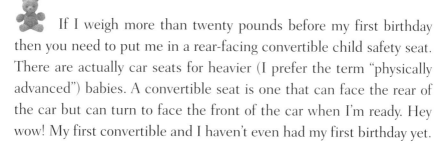

So, you've put me in the car and you've closed the door, but there's one problem. You let me play with your keys. I love pushing those little buttons. I have no idea what they're for, but from the panicked look on your face, you sure do. How come you're knocking on the window and yelling at me?

Never, ever leave me alone in the car! Definition: (Adj) *Not at all . . . no way . . . not ever!* Whether you are running into the store for a quick quart of milk or if I'm sleeping and you don't want me to wake up, if you're running an errand, I'm coming with you. If I'm asleep, then I'll fall back to sleep when you get me to my crib! If removing me from the car makes me cry, believe me, I'll get over it. Crying is in no way dangerous to me, but the dangers of leaving me alone in the car can include: heat stroke, abduction, carbon monoxide poisoning and hypothermia.

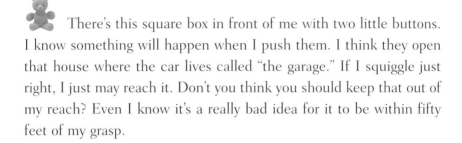

There's this square box in front of me with two little buttons. I know something will happen when I push them. I think they open that house where the car lives called "the garage." If I squiggle just right, I just may reach it. Don't you think you should keep that out of my reach? Even I know it's a really bad idea for it to be within fifty feet of my grasp.

Let's talk fashion. If you don't drive with your hat and mittens on, why should I? Yes, bundle me up in the winter but don't over-bundle.

Note to grown-ups: Heavy clothing on a baby could prevent the harness straps from being snug. If there was an accident the clothes could compress causing the straps to be less secure.

The harness straps on most car seats can be at shoulder level or below. You know, those things that my neck and head rest on. The harness chest clip should be placed at the same level as my armpits.

This keeps the harness straps positioned properly. Remember that each car seat is different, so you must read the instructions because some straps and clips may need to be positioned differently.

Harness straps should fit snugly. Make sure the straps lie in a straight line and don't sag. An adult should not be able to fit more than one finger comfortably between my collarbone and the harness.

Never place any extra cushioning under or behind me. This also prevents harness straps from being snug. You should only use the padding that comes with my safety seat.

Hint: You can place a rolled hand towel around my head and neck for support.

All of that reading you did to me in the womb really paid off. (And you thought I wasn't paying attention.) Here's a phrase that may sound a little complicated: carbon monoxide poisoning. Many folks don't realize it doesn't just happen in the garage. It can happen when

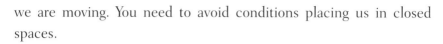

we are moving. You need to avoid conditions placing us in closed spaces.

Note: Once a year, before cold weather begins, check and repair any holes in mufflers or exhaust pipes.

After it snows you need to check something called the tailpipe of our car. Make sure that the snow isn't blocking the tailpipe before you start the car.

Did you know you could buy a car with a sensor system that allows you to know if there is an object directly behind our car? Find out about this because it can save a life one day. (And no, Daddy didn't put me up to hinting about a new car . . . although he did mention this thing called a Ferrari that's very child-friendly.)

Look into buying a car with automatic window sensors. If I accidentally push the window button and put my hand, or worse, in front of the window the sensor will not allow the window to close.

You can never turn your back on me for a split second when I'm outside of the car. I can crawl pretty fast and you don't know where I'm heading. If I drop something under the car, do you know where I'm heading? To get it, of course. You may think those older children who can walk are the only ones who can head for danger in a driveway or parking lot but you're wrong. I'm pretty carefree myself.

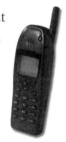

Now that you've learned how to safely install my car seat and to buckle me in, you need to make sure our car seat has not been recalled. I thought this had something to do with my amazing memory but it means that my car seat needs a new part or was found to be unsafe. You can check the Web site of the U.S. Consumer Product Safety Commission, (USCPSC), *www.cpsc.gov,* or National Highway Traffic Safety Administration (NHTSA), *www.nhtsa.dot.gov.*

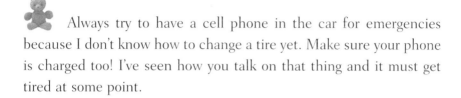

Always try to have a cell phone in the car for emergencies because I don't know how to change a tire yet. Make sure your phone is charged too! I've seen how you talk on that thing and it must get tired at some point.

Make sure you have a safety kit in the car. It's always a good idea to keep Band-Aids, medicines for boo-boos and a blanket to keep me warm. Plus, a bottle and some water or a snack in case we end up getting stuck in traffic or just plain stuck.

I know I'm a distraction, but you need to make sure you keep your eyes on the road so we don't end up with a completely different problem on our hands. I sleep at night and you don't watch me. It's not always necessary to see me. If you feel the need to check me, then let's pull over to a rest stop . . . don't turn around. You need to concentrate on the road.

You know that sun visor you have to protect your eyes from the sun? How about putting one of those things back here as well? I'd like to see the outside world without having to squint.

The safest position for my car seat is usually in the middle seat in the backseat, but only if the car seat fits well in this position. If you need to put me in a seat next to a window, then you need to make sure I can't play with the door and window locks. Do we have those childproof locks? How about turning them on as soon as you fasten your seat belt so you get into the habit of locking them every day. Again . . . just don't lock me in here!

Well, that was a lot of information! I'm tired . . . and you know, my favorite place to fall asleep is safely in the car . . . nighty-night.

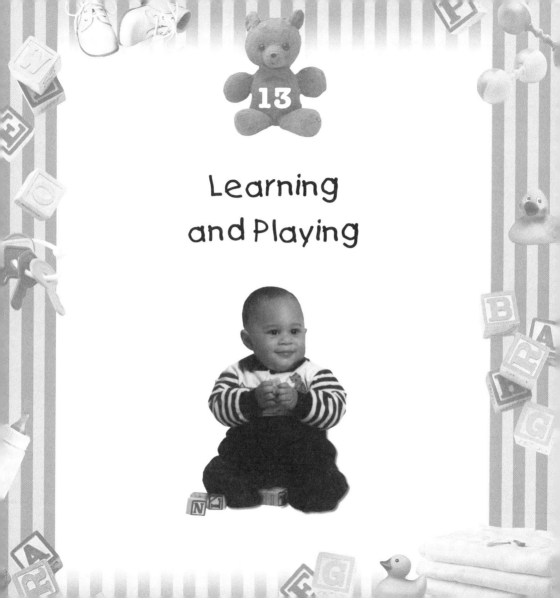

13

Learning
and Playing

For the first few weeks of my life, show me black-and-white toys or toys with brightly contrasting colors. It's what I see best. I know you think pastel and other colorful toys are pretty, but I don't know what pretty is yet; I just know I don't know what color it is. By about three months I'll be able to see all of the colors you are showing me.

In just a few weeks I will be able to tell the difference between different objects, but for now, I can see something that's very important to me . . . your face! At three months, shapes will become clearer, but it will actually take me about six months before I have close to perfect vision.

When I cry, it means I need something. . . . I'm not old enough to fool you until I'm about six months old. Even then, I might not know that I'm fooling you. I don't even know what that means yet. All I know is that when I cry, I need something. I'm probably hungry, wet, gassy, tired, or in need of cuddling or company.

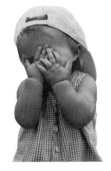

One of the best toys is a burp rag. My mommy takes a clean burp rag and we play peek-a-boo with it. It's a great game. You might see it mentioned a few times in this book because there are many ways to play it.

Make sure squeeze toys do not contain a choker that can detach. If it's possible to swallow it and get it caught in my throat, then I'm going to try and do it.

Are the rattles, teething rings and squeeze toys too large to lodge in my throat? If not, then there is a garbage can with their name on it.

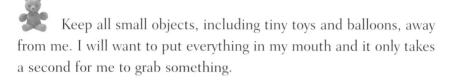

Keep all small objects, including tiny toys and balloons, away from me. I will want to put everything in my mouth and it only takes a second for me to grab something.

Hint: If you think the toy may be too small for me . . . it is.

You may hear a phrase called "tummy time." No, it's not sit-ups for babies. It's allowing me to spend time laying on my side or stomach if—and *ONLY* if—you're watching me the entire time. Switching me to my side and tummy avoids a flattening of my skull and helps my tummy muscles develop. Put me on my tummy for play-time only, not for sleep or naptime!

Note to grown-ups: Wait until my umbilical cord falls off before starting tummy time. Tummy time is spent on the floor, not on high surfaces or a couch because you don't want me rolling off. Keep all unsafe objects away from me and make sure I'm on a clean, safe surface.

When I'm very young, I'll respond to high-pitched sounds and silly noises. If you talk one octave higher using drawn-out vowels I'll be very interested in listening. I may even respond by cooing and kicking my legs.

I will begin learning language by hearing baby-talk. Eventually, when I'm around one, you'll change "horsey" to "horse," and "kitty" to "cat." Time flies and soon you'll wonder what happened to baby-talk.

Start saying my ABC's to me immediately. I need to learn to talk and I will probably learn my vowels first. You can also count to me so I can learn my math. Try counting the spoonfuls as you put them into my mouth or the buttons on my outfit as you button them. I'm not getting into Harvard on my own you know! Waving is an easy trick . . . I can learn that pretty quickly, but don't be surprised if you catch me waving to everything—and I mean everything—I see. It just seems like a fun thing to do.

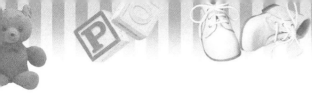

You may want to make the playpen or travel bed more fun for me to play in by adding mattresses or pillows—DON'T! I can actually get caught in the spaces formed between two mattresses. The playpen mattress that comes with the playpen must be snug or I can become trapped and I don't like the sound of that.

Keep older siblings' toys away from me. I know I'm advanced for my age, but I could choke on them.

A playpen is no different than a crib and you should follow the same rules—no soft bedding, no toys with strings or cords and put me to sleep on my back. Think of it as a big bed that I play in . . . the safety rules don't change just because the bed is on the floor and the sides are made of mesh.

You know that mesh stuff that I constantly stick my head up against to look at you through? Make sure the mesh doesn't have any

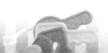

tears, holes or loose threads and is attached securely. You know I am going to try to push myself against it, then through it, and I will eventually use this as a method to escape. You don't want me getting tangled or falling through, do you?

Make sure the top rails of the playpen or travel bed lock into place automatically. If you have to rotate the rails into a locked position then our playpen might have been recalled (that's when something is found to be unsafe to use). I know you like to borrow other people's playpens when we go on trips, but these have become so much better and safer over the years. Please make sure my playpen is safe and we'll both have more fun when I play. Pay attention to product safety and toy recalls. They save lives.

Do not use playpens or travel beds with catch points, such as protruding hardware. More than nine-million older units with protruding hardware have been recalled. That's a lot of spoonfuls, isn't it?

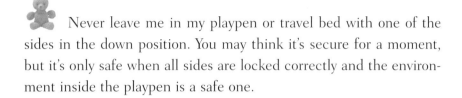

Never leave me in my playpen or travel bed with one of the sides in the down position. You may think it's secure for a moment, but it's only safe when all sides are locked correctly and the environment inside the playpen is a safe one.

I know we've talked about antiques in the past. If I have an older wooden playpen make sure the slats aren't wider than 2⅜ inches. If they are wider, I'm not going in it. You do know that the same goes for a new playpen as well?

Just one more thing about those playpens. I am going to try to escape from those, too. Make sure I don't have any large toys, bumper pads or boxes that I can climb on and make a break for it.

Keep track of consumer product recall information at *www.cpsc.gov* or *www.recalls.gov*.

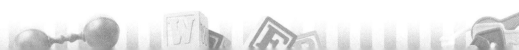

I love to be carried because I love being near you and seeing life from a whole new perspective. When using a back carrier, make sure the leg openings are small enough to prevent me from slipping out but large enough to prevent chafing. If it looks too big then wait a few more weeks; what's your rush anyway? You might as well carry me while I'm still light enough for you to enjoy it.

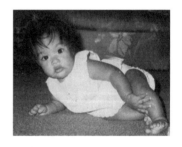

I love peek-a-boo and if you play it with me I will get used to you leaving a room and coming back in again. It's a great way to teach me that you will always come back to me.

Once I begin to stand, you better watch out. I love playing the standing game more than I love playing with my toys. It's fun but when I get tired I'll keep doing it no matter how many times I fall over. Teach me about bending; I keep crashing nose-first to the ground.

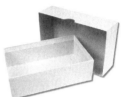

I love boxes and so do all of my friends. If you get a box and it's not too dangerous, let me play with it for a while. I get to bang on it and make noise. Chances are, I'll like the box more than what's inside of it; that's just how things are. The toys are for you and the boxes are for me.

Note to grown-ups: Make sure the edges are smooth and there's no tape or paper I can get ahold of.

Please empty all gift boxes before you give them to me to play with. I can get into all sorts of trouble with wrapping and tissue paper. You know it will only end up in my mouth. And packing "popcorn"? Don't even think about leaving that within twenty feet of me or my playpen. Get rid of every piece!

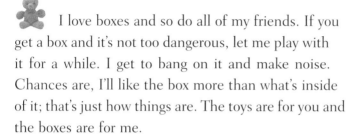

Toys that make music are fun; you can use them to put me to sleep as well. Just remember that the music you teach me to wiggle to should be different than the music you use to put me to sleep.

Don't put all of my toys out at once. It's just as overwhelming for me as it is for you. If you take out only a few at a time it feels like I always have something new to play with. I need to learn to play with one toy at a time. I'm a little too young for that whole "multitasking" idea.

Make sure you take all tags off of my toys. I like to put everything in my mouth. You can't be too careful because I don't know what careful is.

Read to me. You might think I don't understand, and you are right. I probably won't understand for a while, but if you read to me every day, I'll look forward to it when I'm older. The sound of your voice is soothing. I really like when you show me things in picture books.

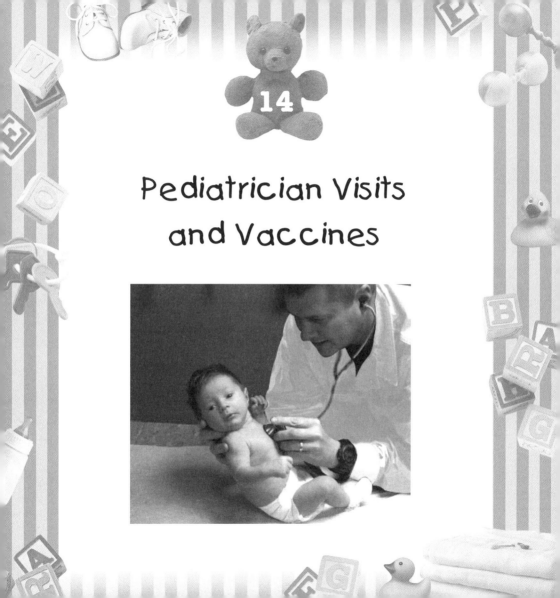

Pediatrician Visits
and Vaccines

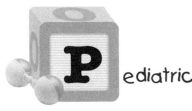 ediatrician Visits

Don't get me all "dolled up" to go to my monthly checkups. The doctor never comes in the room until I'm naked anyway. Just bring me in my PJ's and get me dressed after the doctor is finished poking me.

Bring a bottle or be prepared to nurse whenever we go to the doctor; you never know how long we'll have to wait and there's nothing worse than being starving after a painful shot. I might want a drink and it might help calm me down.

Please bring some toys with you in your diaper bag. So many kids play with those toys at the doctor's office, and those kids aren't all there because they're the picture of perfect health.

Bring extra diapers to every appointment. They always weigh me without my diaper on so you'll need a new diaper after they take me off the scale.

Don't make doctor's appointments on my birthday or yours either. I am going to need shots at almost every appointment, and I don't want to ruin my big day or yours.

Prepare a list of questions to bring with you to my appointments. Chances are I will be fidgety and you won't remember the questions you want to ask the doctor.

See if you can put my top on before they give me my shots because believe me I am going to be upset after those needles and it won't be easy to get me dressed.

Why does the doctor have you and Daddy looking petrified? I'm the one who is about to get stuck with that long prickly thing. Don't worry, we'll all be fine.

If you think I'm not feeling well or you feel at all uncomfortable with the way I look, call the doctor! What can it hurt? So we have a few false alarms; you will have peace of mind and I'll get to know our doctor a little better. Even if it's the middle of the night, it's better to call if you feel something is wrong with me that can't wait till morning.

Vaccines

Shots . . . I hate that word. I know they are important but I'm not sure why. A very important doctor from the Vaccine Education Center at The Children's Hospital of Philadelphia explained it all to me and I am going to do my best to explain it to you. I will even tell you the symptoms of certain diseases and what can happen if you don't vaccinate me for these diseases.

Some vaccines have side effects; you need to measure the risk against the benefit. You have choices about how and when to vaccinate me and you should discuss these in detail with your pediatrician. You will ultimately decide what you feel is right based on all the facts.

The first vaccine is given at birth and it's called hepatitis B. The vaccine for hepatitis A comes when I'm a little older. The order obviously has nothing to do with that song you grown-ups are always trying to teach me. People who have hepatitis B don't always have any symptoms. That means they may have the disease and be walking around with it infecting others around them. Even a toothbrush, washcloth or hand towel can spread this disease. You know how I love to grab for any towel. The symptoms are loss of appetite, vomiting, nausea, fatigue and jaundice (where the skin and whites of the eyes look yellow). It can cause a rapid infection of the liver and can lead to a disease called cirrhosis.

Note: I will get this vaccine again at two months and fifteen months.

The hepatitis B vaccine does have some side effects. It can cause pain, redness and tenderness where I was stuck. It can also, rarely, cause a severe allergic reaction resulting in hives, rash and low blood pressure. If I do have a reaction, it will usually occur within thirty minutes of my shot.

Note: The reactions are rare and not fatal.

At two months I receive several more vaccines. The first is called DTaP. I am scheduled for this shot at two months, four months, six months, eighteen months and between four to six years old.

The "D" in DTaP is for diphtheria, a very serious disease, in which a thick coating forms on the back of the throat, making it difficult to swallow and breathe. A harmful toxin can invade my heart, kidneys and nervous system. The toxin can lead to suffocation, heart failure or paralysis. You should know that diphtheria is something that's very contagious and is spread by coughing and sneezing.

Although diphtheria is a very scary disease you can feel better knowing that only two to five children in the United States get it every year. But, you need to know that fifty thousand cases of diphtheria recently occurred in Russia. As the world is a very small place, unfortunately it only takes one person to bring this disease a little closer to home. The side effects of the diphtheria vaccine are localized pain, redness or tenderness.

 Do you want to know what the "T" in DTaP stands for? It stands for tetanus. Unfortunately, the bacterium for tetanus is found in the soil and there's no way to keep me from playing in the dirt.

The side effects of the vaccine are pain, redness or tenderness where I was stuck. There is a one in a million chance that I will have a severe allergic reaction. If that happens I will get something called hives, a rash or low blood pressure. All of that usually happens within thirty minutes of receiving the vaccine. Now, I don't know about you, but one in a million seems like a small amount to me, but I can't count yet.

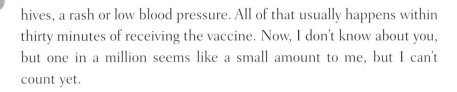 Now it's time to learn what the "P" is in DTaP. The "P" stands for something called pertussis (that's a little big for me). The name isn't one you are likely to forget and the disease is very serious. It causes painful spasms of coughing that make it difficult to breathe, eat or drink. It can lead to something more severe called pneumonia, seizures or even permanent brain damage. I'm not trying to scare you but you need to know all the facts.

Now, the good news is that only about seven thousand cases are reported every year, but as I've already learned, good news is often followed by bad news. The bad news is that most cases aren't reported. A cough that lasts for more than five days in a grown-up has a 5 percent chance of being pertussis. This means that a lot (hundreds of thousands) of grown-ups and teenagers (you know, the people who baby-sit for me) get this disease every year. People like me catch pertussis from young adults who cough.

There can be some side effects to the pertussis vaccine, which occur in one out of every ten-thousand children. I can have pain, redness or swelling where I was stuck. Sometimes it can cause a fever, drowsiness or something called fretfulness (I can become somewhat of a grouch . . . like Oscar on *Sesame Street*). There can be something more serious such as a high fever, inconsolable crying and severe listlessness and lethargy, which typically last a few hours.

There is a very rare bacterium called HIB (that I can pronounce this time). Even though it only affects about 100 to 150 children every year, it can lead to meningitis, which can cause a child to become mentally challenged, deaf, blind or learning disabled. This injection is scheduled for two months, four months, six months and fifteen months.

The HIB injection can cause pain, redness or tenderness where I was stuck or a fever. You need to decide if the side effects are worth the risk. Outbreaks in the U.S. are very rare but it seems to me that you'd rather be safe than sorry on this one.

Here's another one I can almost pronounce: polio. The good news is that polio has been completely eliminated from the United States. The bad news is that there are still outbreaks in India, Africa and parts of Asia. All it takes is one person enjoying a vacation in one of these countries to become infected and come home to the United States. Since it's spread from hand to mouth, it's also very contagious. Polio can cause a mild intestinal infection, but one in every one hundred people infected will be permanently paralyzed. This injection is scheduled for two months, four months, eighteen months and four to six years old.

The name for the polio vaccine is IPV. Do you know what it stands for? I can figure this one out . . . inactivated polio virus. The side effects are pain, redness or tenderness where I was stuck.

Okay . . . this next one is a mouthful. It's called pneumococcus. I wouldn't be attempting to say such a big word if it didn't have such life-threatening potential. It is actually the most common cause of severe bacterial infections of infants and young children.

These can include: meningitis, bloodstream infections, pneumonia, and ear and sinus infections. The vaccine was introduced in the United States in the year 2000. This vaccine is scheduled for two months, four months, six months and fifteen months. Side effects of the pneumococcus vaccine are mild pain, redness and tenderness where I was stuck as well as a mild fever. The side effects are not severe and as you can tell, on this one you'd rather be safe than sorry.

Now it's time for the twelve-month shots. Let's start with something called the MMR. The first "M" stands for measles. Why measles? I don't want 'em . . . so let's call them "your-sles." This shot is also given between four to six years old (I guess that means you are going to stick me again).

Measles! I don't know about you but at first I thought the name seemed harmless. When I heard about what happens to kids who get the measles I decided I want to stay far away from this one. The measles can cause a cough, runny nose, fever, pink eye and a rash that starts on the face and spreads to the rest of the body. It can

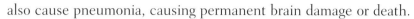

also cause pneumonia, causing permanent brain damage or death.

Only about one hundred children get measles in the United States every year but the bad news is that measles are very contagious and are spread by coughing and sneezing.

The side effects of the vaccine can include pain, redness or tenderness where I am stuck. It can also cause a fever or a rash that occurs eight to ten days after the vaccine is given. The vaccine can also cause a decrease in the number of cells in the bloodstream that are used to help the blood clot.

Mumps, the second "M" . . . another one I can pronounce but want to stay far away from! There are only about five hundred cases in the United States every year but you need to know what could happen. It causes a painful swelling of the glands just below the ear and can lead to meningitis and it can cause permanent hearing loss. The side effects of the vaccine are pain, redness and tenderness where I was stuck.

The "R" stands for rubella. . . . That's a disease? I think I have an aunt by that name. In any case, rubella causes swelling of the glands behind the ear, mild rash and fever. Even though rubella is mild in children, we need to be careful because it can lead to birth defects or be fatal to an unborn baby. That's why you don't want me walking around with rubella as I meet a lot of pregnant women.

The possible side effects with the rubella vaccine can include some pain, redness or tenderness where I was stuck. It can also cause a short-lived swelling of the joints (arthritis). This reaction is only temporary.

Another twelve-month shot is to prevent chicken pox. If I get chicken pox I will get blisters, a fever and I'll have fierce itching that will last for days. Yes, once I've had it, I won't get it again, but why make me suffer? Here's some chicken pox trivia: How did chicken pox get its name? No, it has nothing to do with crossing the road. The blisters produced by the chicken pox virus are said to resemble a chicken after it's been plucked. Take the experts' word for it and don't try that at home.

Chicken pox is more than just a few bumps. I can get three hundred to five hundred blisters and it can infect my lungs, leading to pneumonia. In more severe cases, it can infect my brain (encephalitis) and cause severe skin infections.

The side effects of the vaccine are pain, redness or tenderness where I was stuck. Some children will develop blisters after receiving the vaccine but that number is fewer than 5 percent.

Note to grown-ups: A very small amount of people can get chicken pox twice. It is almost always a one-time illness. If you get a mild case when you are under a year you have a higher chance of getting it again.

Hepatitis A. Remember we learned about hepatitis B earlier in the chapter? Just like hepatitis B, people don't always have symptoms, which include loss of appetite, vomiting (I'm familiar with that one), nausea, fatigue and jaundice. It can be severe, causing rapid infection of the liver and death.

Hepatitis A is spread through contaminated food or water. Some states have a higher rate of infection than others and those are the

ones where it's recommended the vaccine should be given. These include Arizona, Alaska, Oregon, New Mexico, Utah, Washington, Oklahoma, South Dakota, Nevada, California and Idaho. (Not bad for an infant, huh? Just don't ask me to name their capitals.)

The side effects of the vaccine are pain, warmth or swelling where I was stuck and some children will get a headache (that happens about 5 percent of the time).

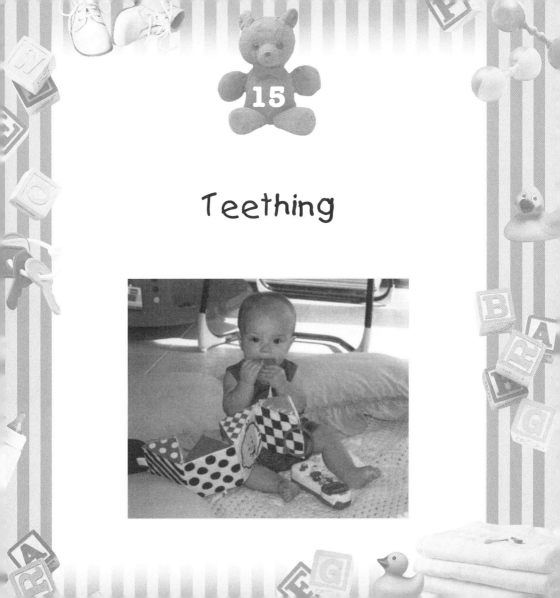

15

Teething

Believe me . . . this is a lot harder for me than it is for you. There's a good chance I am going to wake up in the middle of the night and I'll probably be gnawing on my hands all day.

I love teething rings but make sure you put them in the refrigerator and not the freezer. You wouldn't believe how many parents make this mistake. Can you chew on an ice cube? I can't. There are some teething rings made for the freezer but you may want to stick to the softer kind.

Don't give me a frozen bagel or an ice cube to help my teething. You might not think so, but I could choke on it. After I suck on it for a little while, a frozen bagel will eventually defrost.

You can make me feel better by gently massaging my gums with one of your nice, clean fingers. It makes sense to me; I'm always ready for a nice massage.

How about a Popsicle? Just don't let a big chunk fall into my mouth. Only let me suck on it for a few minutes. It is soooo soooothing. Try not to give me bright red-colored ones. I will be wearing whatever color you give me and so will my clothes. Use a bib and be ready for a mess. A big mess.

If you are really worried about Popsicle stains put me in the bathtub. I'll be nice and clean and my teeth will be nice and numb before night-night.

Okay, so you've never seen a baby drool so much. I can't help it. It could be worse—you could've gotten a puppy. You are going to need extra burp cloths so always have them handy.

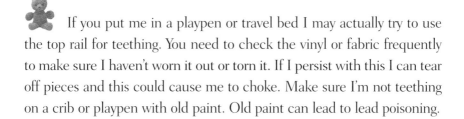

If you put me in a playpen or travel bed I may actually try to use the top rail for teething. You need to check the vinyl or fabric frequently to make sure I haven't worn it out or torn it. If I persist with this I can tear off pieces and this could cause me to choke. Make sure I'm not teething on a crib or playpen with old paint. Old paint can lead to lead poisoning.

You can give me a baby toothbrush to teethe on. This way I can actually clean my new teeth and feel some relief at the same time. But no toothpaste please, because I'll get a tummy ache. Don't let me crawl around with a toothbrush because I could poke myself.

I'm not allowed to sleep with teething rings!

Okay, you've tried everything—you've picked me up, cuddled me, walked the floor—and I'm still crying? Well, imagine how I feel! I'm the one cutting a tooth here. Try freezing a washcloth and giving it to me to suck on.

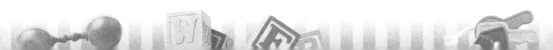

Now that I have teeth, you need to know how to clean them. Don't forget to use baby toothpaste because your toothpaste contains too much fluoride for me. Start early—I want to show off my smile.

If I'm still a little too young for a toothbrush, take a piece of gauze and wipe my teeth with it. Make sure it stays in your hand and doesn't end up in my mouth!

Have plenty of diaper rash cream ready. No, I'm not going to rub it on my sore gums. When I teethe, I produce more saliva that travels through my digestive system leading to all sorts of new developments. There is a chance that this could cause me to get a diaper rash. Believe me, if I get a diaper rash on top of this new tooth, you and Daddy are going to start getting that stressed-out look on your faces again.

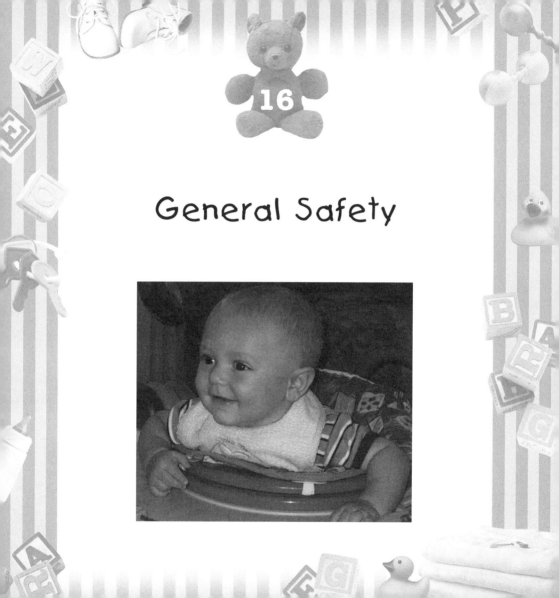

General Safety

S trollers

Old strollers can be risky. Some of these old strollers don't have safe harnesses. I can actually slip and become trapped in the leg openings. Please make sure the restraints work properly. I wouldn't expect you to use a broken seat belt in a car.

It's called a stroller . . . not a bed. If I do fall asleep in it, make sure it's not in the reclining position. I can squiggle to the front and get caught between the hand-rest and the front edge of the seat.

A stroller is a chair on wheels, so always fasten me in. Make sure the buckles are sturdy and durable and that I fit snugly.

I know you think that hand-rest on the stroller is a great place to put your bags but you can actually make me tip over. Sorry, you'll have to hold them or put them underneath the stroller.

My stroller has brakes? Can I use them? How about if you use them! Make sure they are easy for you to operate. Even if they are on, you can't leave me alone in here . . . awake or asleep!

One more thing about strollers: Keep me away from them when you are folding them. My fingers and hands can get caught. It sounds pretty scary to me. I guess that's why they are called strollers and not toys . . . don't let me play with my stroller.

Water Hazards

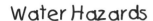

Can you believe I can drown in a five-gallon bucket of water? We have plenty of those around for that housework I see you doing. To me, five gallons of water is an Olympic-sized pool. It won't tip over if I fall into it; I will just get stuck in it. So don't leave one around unless there's a lifeguard on duty.

When you are doing yard work, never leave a bucket containing even an inch or two of liquid unattended. When you finish using a bucket, always empty it immediately and bring it inside. If it's left outside it can collect rainwater. Always put it away and keep it out of reach, especially my reach. How hard is that?

Yes, a toilet can be very dangerous. My head is heavier than the rest of my body and I can fall headfirst into the toilet if I decide to explore. Get a lock—you don't want me playing in there anyway.

Electrical Outlets

Use safety plugs to cover electrical outlets. I like sticking my fingers in everything. Did you know it's even more fun to stick my toys into those holes? Who knows what can happen? I don't.

I know you think I'm too smart to stick anything in an electrical outlet, but I'm also very curious. It looks like an interesting puzzle to me and I want to see what I can fit in there.

Extension cords are dangerous as well. If I get the extension part anywhere near my mouth I can get quite a burn. It's like giving me a giant electrical rope to play with. If you must use them, try wrapping the ends that connect together with electrical tape and try not to use them in my playroom or a room I visit frequently.

Safety Gates

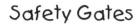 Make sure all safety gates have a pressure bar or other fastener that will resist pressure when I push on it. If you leave me behind a gate, I will do everything I can to knock it down.

Make sure the openings in a safety gate are too small to entrap my head. I will try to stick my head through this fence as soon as possible. Make sure I can't do it.

Check the safety gate to make sure it's secure. I will try to push on it and it can become loose. You know how much I want to figure out how to open this thing.

Why did you only put a safety gate at the top of the stairs and not the bottom? Don't you want to stop me from going up as well as going down? We need safety gates at the bottom and the top of the stairs!

Have you installed a childproof latch on the outside of the bathroom door to prevent me from entering? Better yet, put one on so I don't get locked in. Don't wait for the inevitable. Some rooms need to be off-limits to me.

Pacifiers

Do not attach ribbon, string cord or yarn to a pacifier. I can easily get tangled in those things or they can cut off my circulation.

Is the pacifier shield large enough and firm enough not to fit into my mouth? If not, then you're off to the store to buy a new one. By the way, make sure there are ventilation holes on this as well.

Make sure my pacifier can't separate into small pieces. You've seen how much I enjoy it; it better be sturdy. Check them often for tears and holes. If they are worn out, throw them away. I'm sure you know where to find more.

Do not tie the pacifier around my neck. I'm sure you can figure out the reason. Let's expand that—don't tie *anything* around my neck! It seems obvious to me.

Choking/Poisoning

If I accidentally ingest something I shouldn't, call the Poison Control Center at 1-800-222-1222.

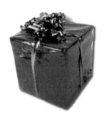

There's a poison we can't see or smell but it's deadly. It's called carbon monoxide. You should have a carbon monoxide detector in the house to protect all of us.

Keep all plastic wrappers and bags out of my reach. Look around the house for any bags lying around that I can put over my head. Even my mattress comes in a plastic wrapper . . . a rather large one, I may add. Throw it away! As quickly as plastic wrappers enter the house, they should leave as well!

During holiday time pick up and throw away all wrapping, strings and bows. I'm very fast and I can easily put a plastic bag over my head or paper in my mouth while you're busy unwrapping those pretty gifts.

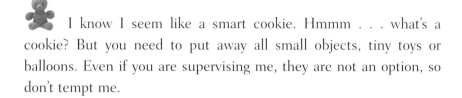

I know I seem like a smart cookie. Hmmm . . . what's a cookie? But you need to put away all small objects, tiny toys or balloons. Even if you are supervising me, they are not an option, so don't tempt me.

All medicines and cleaning products need to be locked away and kept in containers with safety caps. If I somehow get my hands on one of those containers (which I know you won't let happen), I shouldn't be able to open it. Never leave medicine—mine or yours—sitting on a counter even for a minute. I'm faster than you think!

Okay, so you think you've locked away all of the hazards, but did you remember to put away the matches and lighters? After you light a candle, the fireplace or the grill, put away the lighting device. I know you won't let me near any of those things you've just lit but you have to hide the matches as well. They seem very interesting and I'm watching that little light appear and I want to do it.

Move refrigerator magnets out of my reach or remove them altogether. I don't know what those things are for but they seem to be just the right size for my mouth.

Do you always put the cap back on medicine bottles? What's the point of a childproof cover if you don't use it? How about covering the toothpaste when you're finished? I'm not trying to be a neat freak. I just know that I can choke on the cap, so you need to put these back in place and keep them far away from me.

I know we received tons of rattles as gifts, but are they safe? Make sure they can't become lodged in my mouth and that no pieces can actually separate from the rattle. If you have any doubts take it away from me and contact the U.S. Consumer Product Safety Commission. This is something I put in my mouth; let's make sure it stays in one piece.

Be sure to replace or repair any loops in window blind cords. Blinds made since November 2000 have no loops, so consider buying newer, safer blinds.

Drawstrings look cute but they can get caught on play equipment, furniture or my crib. You don't need to avoid clothes with them altogether; you can just remove them from my jackets and sweatshirts. Did you know they make clothes with buttons, snaps and Velcro? What will they think of next?

Lead Poisoning

Did you know that lead-based paint in old homes is the number one cause of lead poisoning? Lead poisoning can lead to learning, hearing and behavioral problems. Lead can harm my kidneys, brain and other organs. A simple blood test can confirm lead poisoning. Children should be tested at twelve months with a follow-up at twenty-four months.

If my blood level is shown to be elevated for lead, our local health department will visit our home to help find the source of the lead and tell us how we can reduce our risk. Some of the ways will include getting rid of the lead paint, checking the soil surrounding our house and washing areas frequently.

What's the likelihood of us having lead-based paint? The older the home, the higher the chances. If our paint is peeling, chipping, chalking or cracking, it could be hazardous to me. Personally, I don't like the sound of that. Even if the paint on our home doesn't have a single flaw, it can be harmful to me if it's something I chew. What's the likelihood of me chewing on something? One hundred percent. Is that a lot?

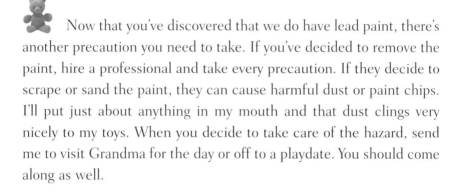

Now that you've discovered that we do have lead paint, there's another precaution you need to take. If you've decided to remove the paint, hire a professional and take every precaution. If they decide to scrape or sand the paint, they can cause harmful dust or paint chips. I'll put just about anything in my mouth and that dust clings very nicely to my toys. When you decide to take care of the hazard, send me to visit Grandma for the day or off to a playdate. You should come along as well.

Hey, it's nice out here in the yard and I love to dig in the soil. Be careful: Our soil could be contaminated if lead-based paint from our house flakes or peels and gets into the soil.

A job! What's that? Is that where people are rushing off to all day? People at certain jobs can be exposed to lead. If someone in our family works in construction, plumbing, painting or auto repair, they should shower and change into fresh clothes and shoes before

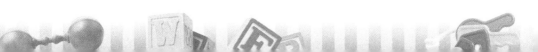

coming home. There are other jobs that could expose people to lead, so you need to find out if it's a job that someone in our family does. These work clothes need to be washed separately.

Common Poisonous Plants

Aloe vera	Chalice vine	Jerusalem cherry
Amaryllis	Croton	Kafir lily
Angel's trumpet	Cyclamen	Lantana
Angel's wings	Crown of thorns	Narcissus—daffodil
Aralia	Devil's ivy	Peace Lily
Asparagus fern	Dumb cane	Philodendron
Australian umbrella tree	Elephant's ear	Poinsettia (can cause skin irritation)
Azalea	Eucalyptus	
Balsam pear	Flamingo flower	Schefflera
Bird of paradise flower	Heart-leaf Philodendron	Snow-on-the-mountain
Caladium	Hyacinth	Spider lily
Candelabra cactus	Hydrangea	Swiss cheese plant
Castor bean	Irises	
	Java Bean	

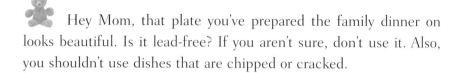

Hey Mom, that plate you've prepared the family dinner on looks beautiful. Is it lead-free? If you aren't sure, don't use it. Also, you shouldn't use dishes that are chipped or cracked.

Burns

To avoid burns when you are bathing me, always turn on the cold water first and turn off the hot water first. Your hands should always touch the water before it touches me and NEVER put me directly under the faucet. Don't put me anywhere near the water until the water is a safe temperature.

Note: Rather than risk a burn, check our water temperature to see if it is more than 120°F (49°C). You can call the company that provides the fuel to heat our water. Gas, electric and oil companies will reset the temperatures on hot water heaters to below the scalding level if asked to do so.

If we live in an apartment, you can call the superintendent of the building to explain that water hotter than 49°C can burn me. He or she may be able to lower the water temperature. Or you may be able to put an anti-scald device on our taps.

Do we have radiators, a gas fireplace or baseboard heaters in our home? Make sure to keep me at a distance from heaters and devices that get too hot and could cause a potential burn or injury. I don't know what those things are but they look like something I could use to help pull myself up.

Fire Safety

To protect us from a fire, make sure we have a working smoke detector in our house. You can also buy a heat detector for the kitchen (this doesn't take the place of a smoke detector). Check the batteries once a month to make sure they are working and change them regularly.

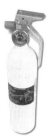

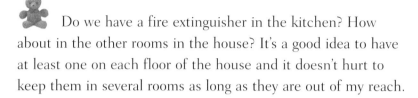 Do we have a fire extinguisher in the kitchen? How about in the other rooms in the house? It's a good idea to have at least one on each floor of the house and it doesn't hurt to keep them in several rooms as long as they are out of my reach.

Now that we are well equipped with fire extinguishers, do you know how to use them? Make sure you read the instructions ahead of time. If we have an emergency, you won't have time to start reading the instructions.

Note to grown-ups: There are different types of fire extinguishers for different types of fires . . . the fire extinguisher you keep in the garage may not be the same as the one you keep in the kitchen.

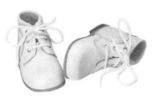

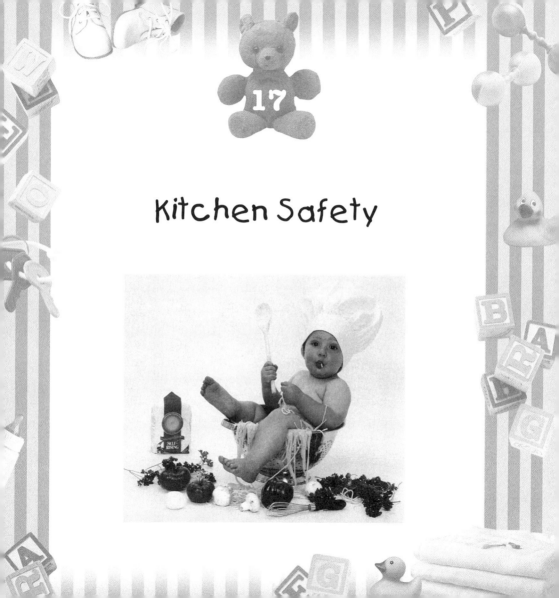

Kitchen Safety

The kitchen is a very dangerous room. Once I start crawling, you need to think about getting safety locks for the lower cabinets. You keep all sorts of cleaners and supplies in there that you don't want me getting my hands on.

You should get into the habit of using the back burners of the stove and turning all pot handles toward the wall. . . . Once I'm able to pull myself up, you'd be surprised what I can reach. I see you playing with those pots and I want to do the same. You've heard the horror stories—I don't want to be one.

You can buy covers for the knobs on the stove, making them impossible for me to turn. I don't know what those knobs do . . . I am just waiting for the noise to start and the lights to flash, just like the rest of my toys. I know something always happens when I turn a knob.

I might love to play with the pots and pans on the kitchen floor safely away from the stove because I want to be where you are working. I need to be where you can see me and where I can talk to you. You can keep me in the kitchen with you but you must keep me safe.

Don't leave the oven door open even if it's cooled and turned off. If I crawl on the open oven door, it can tip over on me. It's never too early to talk to me about staying away from the stove.

If I ever get burned, don't panic, please! Quick action is needed and you'll have to stay cool. Flush the burn with cold water immediately and keep running cool water over it. If the burn is larger than the size of a quarter, or blisters, call the doctor right away.

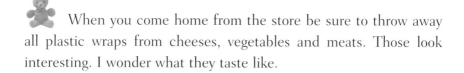

When you come home from the store be sure to throw away all plastic wraps from cheeses, vegetables and meats. Those look interesting. I wonder what they taste like.

What are those shiny things you are using to cut your food into little pieces? I'd like to see those, so keep them out of my reach. Don't forget to do this at restaurants, too.

Did you know dishwasher detergent is one of the most poisonous substances in the house? If you spill even the tiniest bit of powder, clean it up immediately.

The dishwasher is a very dangerous place. Never empty or load the dishwasher while I'm in the room. If I fall into it there is nothing except jagged spikes to break my fall. Just wait till I'm napping or in my high chair to empty the dishwasher. It looks like an interesting place to visit and I'm just waiting for my chance to explore the inside of that machine.

When you empty your groceries, keep all dangerous items out of my reach. I know that box of foil looks like a fun thing for me to play with, but it has jagged edges.

That garbage pail looks like a lot of fun. I keep seeing you throw things in there and I want to try it, too. I might even find something fun to play with. I have no idea what garbage is, but it looks pretty neat. I think you better get a pail with a cover that you can put a baby lock on as well.

It's time to clean out under the kitchen sink. This is usually the cabinet that needs the most protection from me. Look at all of the labels. If you have any chemicals without labels, throw them away. You aren't going to use them anyway. You need to be aware of every chemical you have in the house and only keep what you really intend to use. The best idea . . . find another place to store all chemicals.

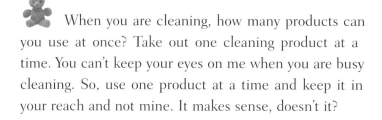

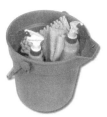

When you are cleaning, how many products can you use at once? Take out one cleaning product at a time. You can't keep your eyes on me when you are busy cleaning. So, use one product at a time and keep it in your reach and not mine. It makes sense, doesn't it?

Always keep all household chemicals and cleaners in their original containers. Even though you feel these are well out of my reach you need to be prepared in case of accidental poisoning. The poison control center will ask you the name of the substance I ingested.

Note to grown-ups: Lock up all poisonous substances. If you aren't sure if something is poisonous, it gets locked up as well.

If I accidentally ingest a poisonous substance, you need to call the poison control center immediately. Don't give me syrup of Ipecac or force me to throw up until you call the poison control center to find out the safest way to help me.

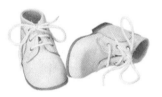

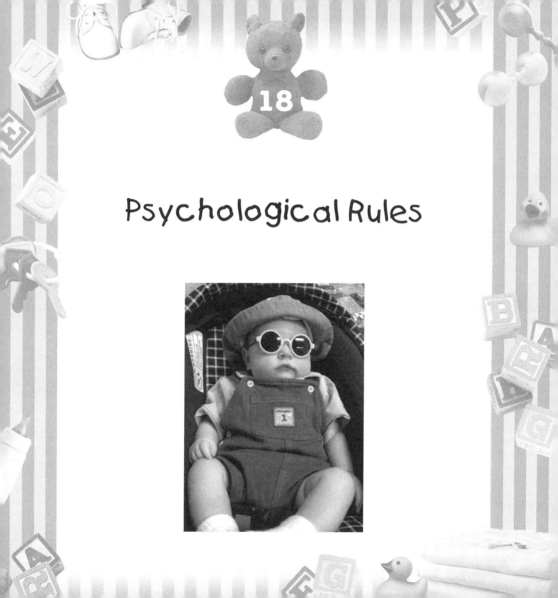

Psychological Rules

18

"**Y**ou're going to spoil that baby!" Why does every family we know, including ours, have a relative who thinks a newborn like me can be spoiled? I'm too young to be spoiled. When I cry, it's because I need something—like to nurse, have a bottle, a diaper change, a burp or you. . . . I'm not crying for a toy. Newborns can't fool you so don't let anyone think I'm playing games. . . . I don't even know what a game is.

I'm just a few weeks old and I'm crying. Do you know what I need? I may be cold, hungry, tired or I may not be feeling well. For starters, try feeding, burping, changing and rocking me or playing with me. Please, not all at the same time! Soon you will learn my cries and figure out exactly what I need.

Some new mommies and daddies tend to become frantic when they hear their baby crying. I sense all of your moods and emotions. If you calmly try to figure out what I need, then I will respond in the same way—calmly.

Don't become agitated when you can't calm me down. Just give me some time. I may not even know exactly why I'm crying. Wait a bit. If nothing else, I'll cry myself to sleep, and that's okay, too.

Try your best not to argue or raise your voice in front of me. If I grow up around arguing adults, then I'll become one myself. Remember, children follow by example. My childhood is not just what I make of it; it's what you make of it as well.

Read to me! You may think I'm too young to understand but you'd be surprised at what I retain. If you read to me as a baby, I'll want you to continue when I'm a toddler. Wouldn't it be nice to have some quiet reading time together every night? If it's what I learn now, it's the routine I will be used to as I grow up.

If you don't want me to touch something, take it away from me. Let me see that if I touch it, it will disappear. I really hate when this happens but I'll learn that it's not mine.

Music, Maestro . . . I mean Mother. Some music would be nice. If you play some soft, soothing music to me it may calm me down when I'm crying. Sing some songs to me as well. I am comfortable with familiarity. When I'm in a new environment or I feel overwhelmed, you might be able to calm me down with a familiar song, saying or toy.

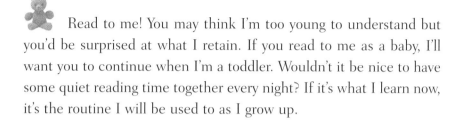

Okay, I'm four months old now. I am beginning to catch on that when I cry, you come to my rescue. I'm still not old enough to fool you, but get ready, because I'm getting smarter.

I'm six months old and I've become very tricky. (I've pretty much gotten you trained by now.) I like to play this game where I cry and you let me play rather than putting me in my crib. I need to learn that when you put me in the crib, I'm there to stay, whether I fall asleep or not! The crib is the safest place for me to be, so put me in there during nap time. Even if I don't sleep, I'll learn that nap time is nap time and playtime is playtime.

If you constantly say no to me, don't be surprised if it's one of my first words. Learn other words or tones of voice to stop me from what I'm doing. Distracting me with something I'm allowed to play with is another option.

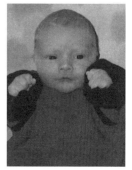

It's much harder to teach me right from wrong and definitely requires tremendous patience . . . but don't give in to my crying when there is a lesson to be learned. We'll both have an easier time of things later if I learn early on that you mean what you say and say what you mean. It will be easier for me to learn the household rules if they're consistent.

If I keep getting myself into trouble with your valuables, try to distract me with something I'm allowed to play with. Show me a new toy and continue to take away the things you don't want me to touch. Sooner or later I'll realize right from wrong. Hey, I may seem advanced but I'm just a baby.

Don't be upset if my food winds up on the floor. You probably haven't realized it yet but food on the floor means I'm done eating and I think it would be fun to play with my peas and carrots. Developmentally, it fascinates me to watch things fall to the floor out of my little hands. A guy named Sir Isaac Newton had the same fascination and look where it got him!

An ounce of love is the most valuable medicine in the world. You can teach me right from wrong and how to respond by showing me with love. Teach me that if I do something correct, I will be rewarded. If I do something wrong like throwing my toys, take them away until I calm down.

You may feel nervous or even guilty the first time you hire a baby-sitter to take care of me. I'm sure you will call the sitter ten times. I wonder who she's sitting . . . you or me!

It's not enough to tell the sitter where everything is located; you should show the sitter as well. Don't take it for granted that the sitter can find my PJ's or my favorite toy. Even more important, you may think you've put a bottle in the fridge, not

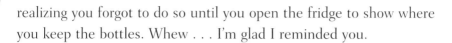

realizing you forgot to do so until you open the fridge to show where you keep the bottles. Whew . . . I'm glad I reminded you.

You need to check the references of every sitter, nanny, care-giver and child-care center. Not only are you ensuring you're leaving me in good hands, you are giving yourself peace of mind. You'll feel a lot better leaving me with someone else if you've double- and triple-checked their qualifications and references.

When you hire a baby-sitter, you need to do everything you can to make it a positive experience for you. If you are afraid you may forget to tell the baby-sitter something or that the sitter may forget something, write it down. Be sure to include all emergency numbers, numbers you can be reached at and even the number of a neighbor. Now that she has the numbers to everyone in the state, tell her never to take her eyes off of me, and enjoy your night out.

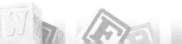

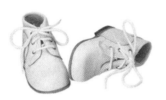

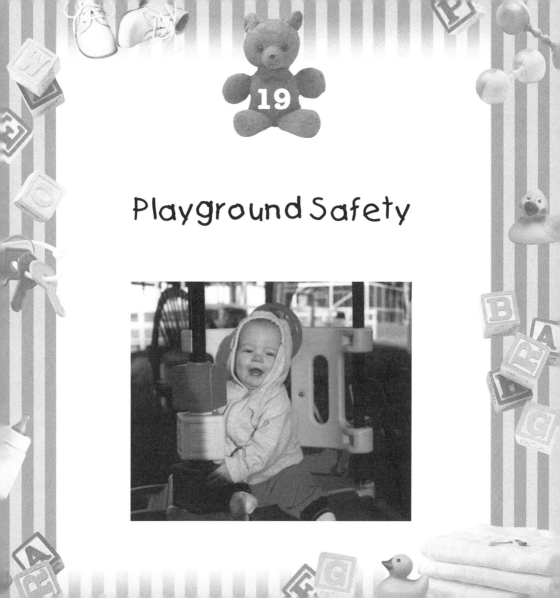

19

Playground Safety

Now it's time for me to practice my letters and give you some playground safety tips all at the same time (not bad for a newborn). Here are the ABC's of playground safety.

A is for Age

Did you know that as of this publishing, there are no playground equipment standards for children under two years old? That means the swings, slides and climbing equipment weren't built for me. They were built for my older friends and siblings. But, for the first time, a standard for play equipment for children ages four months to two years old will be published in 2004, by the American Society for Testing and Materials (ASTM). For now, I'll share some advice for my older friends and siblings, and for you to remember when you take me to the playground when I'm a big kid.

B is for Bay

Did you know that a park or school should only have two swings for each bay/structure supporting the swing? Old playground equipment will have four swings on a structure. Most kids I know like to walk between the swings or behind them. Make sure that the area is safe. Two swings to an area, please!

C is for Chains

Check the chains and S-hooks on the swings. If anything is rusting, open or breaking, it must be replaced. Do not buy the chains or hooks from anyone other than the swing-set company. Some swing-set chains are covered with soft colored plastic. Do you know what's going on under that plastic? You better check for rust there, too! I know it's a pain, but imagine the pain I'll be in from a fall.

Here's some good info for you: The chains at the public playground should be changed every year or when the manufacturer says

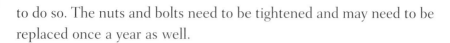

to do so. The nuts and bolts need to be tightened and may need to be replaced once a year as well.

D is for Digging

I love digging in the sandbox but I have no idea what's really in that sand. Keep our sandbox at home clean by covering it. Care centers should cover their sandboxes too. It know it's a little bit more difficult to know what's really in the sand at the park; but you can call the parks department and ask them to clean the sand. Do it for me.

E is for Exploring

Some parks and playgrounds have cute little houses for me to explore. These can be a lot of fun, just be sure that the older kids can't climb on top of my house. An older child may fall and not only hurt himself but could fall on top of me. Look carefully inside for litter or even insect nests first before I explore.

F is for Fall

Falls to surfaces are responsible for more than 70 percent of the injuries in playgrounds. Just remember, when I'm a preschooler, I'll need twelve inches of loose fill for equipment up to six feet in height. Do you know what loose fill is? I didn't either. It's wood fiber, pea gravel, sand or shredded rubber. Don't you remember how painful it was to fall off a swing? If you are thinking of getting me a swing set when I'm older, please put it over a foot of loose fill.

G is for Grass

You must never put a child on a playset that is placed over grass. When I'm a preschooler, equipment must be over a surface of loose fill at least twelve inches deep for equipment up to six feet high.

Now that you know what loose fill is, it shouldn't be a problem.

Note: If you decide to use a synthetic surface for our home equipment, the manufacturer should make recommendations of the depth of their products depending on equipment height. Wow, that lingo is totally over my head, but I'm confident you'll know what it means.

H is for Hidden Hazards

There are many hidden hazards in parks and playgrounds. We may even have some of these hazards on our home swing set. These include broken glass or metal pieces, or playground design that creates congestion, allowing me to collide or fall onto one of my playmates. Metal equipment in open sunlight without a protective surface to prevent my tushie or other important parts from burns is dangerous. Areas without fencing can allow me to run in front of cars. Always be on the lookout for these hidden hazards.

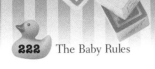

I is for Injury

 Did you know that 40 percent of playground injuries are related to inadequate supervision? There's that percent word again. You grown-ups are awfully preoccupied with that word. You should always have your eyes on me when I'm at the playground. Not only do you need to watch for potential hazards such as damaged equipment, you need to watch for speeding targets.

Hint: I'm referring to the other children at the playground. The children who loaded up on simple carbohydrates (SUGAR!) just before coming to the playground! You know the kids I'm talking about . . . the ones who think the playground is the Indianapolis 500.

J is for Jump

If the climbing equipment has a platform, it should be surrounded with a guardrail or protective barrier so I don't fall or decide to jump. The height of the barrier depends on my age and the height of the platform. When I'm younger (which I'll be for a while), the guardrails and protective barriers should be at least twenty-nine inches high. For bigger or school-aged kids, they should have barriers that are at least thirty-eight inches high.

K is for Kids

Our equipment at home needs a different kind of attention than the one at the park or school. The equipment at the park was built to withstand much more activity. (That means that they are prepared for hundreds of kids a day. You only have to be prepared for my friends, my siblings and me.) If you are concerned about the equipment at the park, call the parks department in our town.

L is for Labels

The equipment at the park needs to be labeled so you know what equipment my friends and siblings can play on (and me when

I'm old enough). You can't put a two-year-old on a piece of equipment that is made for a ten-year-old. Children develop differently and I'm sure you know that a toddler can't possibly do the same things as a child more than twice his/her age. Just remember, there are twelve-year-olds playing at our park. Do you really think I should be on the same equipment? Our park should have different playing areas for preschoolers and school-age children and should have signs on the equipment to tell you which is which . . . so you don't get confused AND SO I DON'T GET HURT!

M is for Monkey Bars

You might remember monkey bars from when you were a kid, or can't you remember back that far? These structures are made of pipe and look like a vertical square with bars on the inside. I should NEVER be allowed to play on them. These should be removed from playgrounds. It's okay for me to play on horizontal ladders when I'm in kindergarten.

N is for National Program for Playground Safety

The National Program for Playground Safety is a group that monitors and advocates for playground safety. They have lots of cool information you can find at *www.playgroundsafety.org.*

O is for Old

Just like people, playground equipment can show wear and tear. Since the play set we use at home isn't made to withstand constant use like playground structures, when you think our play set is too old, don't donate it to a care center or school . . . take it to the dump.

P is for Protection

Even if the park has a lot of shade, cover me with sunscreen and dress me in protective clothing when you take me outside for any length of time. As a newborn, though, help me avoid direct sun until the doctor says I'm old enough for sunscreen and tells you which kind is safe.

Q is for Quick

We toddlers can be quick. Most importantly, children need adult supervision at all times. No matter what you think, a child cannot be left unsupervised at a play-ground for even a moment. You know I'm just waiting for that split second that you turn your back so I can have the kind of fun that always gets me into serious trouble.

R is for Rust

Replace rusting nuts and bolts from our swing set at home. Please don't go to the local hardware store or one of those large chain stores for these pieces. Those stores don't provide the same nuts and bolts as the company who sold us the playground equipment. The

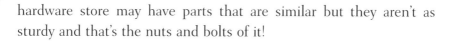

hardware store may have parts that are similar but they aren't as sturdy and that's the nuts and bolts of it!

S is for Speak Up

I know you can speak up because I hear you doing it at home! Remember that I deserve a safe public park and playground and you shouldn't feel bad about demanding it! You need to know that you must take matters into your own hands. If something isn't safe, call someone and make sure they change it. How do you know if something is a danger to me? Two things: information and parental instinct! If you think something is hazardous, it probably is! You can probably find the phone number of the parks department in the phone book, a sign at the park or by calling our local city hall.

T is for Trees

All playgrounds need to be inspected for tree safety. A dead tree or branch can fall and be extremely dangerous. If you see trees that need to be cut down or trimmed, call your park service immediately.

Important hint: Please inspect the trees around our home and any places where I play or if we go camping as well. Trees are a hidden danger that I need you to take very seriously. If a tree or branch is dead, remove it immediately.

U is for Underneath

If I could get hurt from falling onto grass, imagine what could happen if I fall onto a harder surface such as asphalt, concrete or packed dirt. If playground equipment is placed over a hard surface the rule is simple: No kids are allowed to play on it. Let me give you some examples of what you can use underneath a swing set: wood fiber, pea gravel, sand, shredded rubber, rubber tiles, mats or poured surfaces.

Note: If you visit any indoor play places, the same rules apply: They must have mats that have passed something known as the ASTM standards.

V is for Vertical Climber

All tree branches need to be removed from the first seven feet of a tree. Those older kids know the trick of vertical climbing and they will try almost anything. Leave it to us kids to ignore the expensive playground equipment that is safety approved and opt for the dangerous tree that is a potential wonderland of injury. If it looks unsafe, tell someone who can do something to fix this hazard.

W is for Wood

Did you know that swing seats shouldn't be made of wood or metal? They should have soft seats and can be made of rubber. I've heard tales of kids being badly injured who run in front of one of those fast-moving objects. A wood or metal swing can be very harmful to a little head like mine.

X marks the spot

Don't just bring my tricycle or bicycle to the park thinking it's a safe place for me to ride. You need to make sure I can't get hurt by cars or other kids. Some parks have a specific spot for little riders. They actually have cute little paths for me to follow. Don't allow me on those paths unless they are out of the zones in which children can fall. You don't need to bring a ruler to the park. If it doesn't look safe, don't put me near it.

Note: When I'm ready to ride a tricycle, be sure I wear a helmet. It should DEFINITELY be removed before I am allowed to play on playground equipment.

Y is for You

I know you think you can sit and watch me and everything will be all right, but I'm very unpredictable at my age. The most important key to my safety is you! One thing you can count on is that I love to do the opposite of what you want me to do. You'd better hold my hand while walking past potentially dangerous playground equipment and be alert, because you can bet I'll do everything to try to escape from your kung fu grip.

Z is for Zone

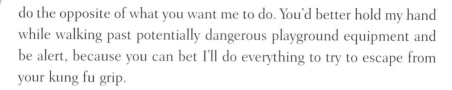 A "use zone" is the area around the swing set should I decide to jump off the swing when I'm bigger and need a safe place to land. The use zone is twice the height of the swing. So, if the swing set is seven feet high, the use zone is fourteen feet from the front of the swing seat and fourteen feet from the back of the seat. This needs to be covered with twelve inches of loose fill. It's a safe bet that I'll jump at some point so make it safe for me. By the way, this jumping off the swing business is only one element of my preoccupation with flying, which will cause you numerous gray hairs and is one of the "perks" of parenthood.

Let me tell you about other use zones. Stationary equipment such as slides have use zones too. These use zones are the surfacing

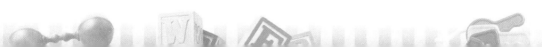

below the equipment. For example, there must be six feet of suitable surfacing all around the slide piece and at the end of a slide that is four feet long.

If the slide is longer, then remember this: The use zone is the height of the platform plus four feet. So, when I'm older if you put me on an eight-foot slide . . . there'd better be twelve feet of cushioning to break my fall at the end of the slide and six feet all around the structure. (And you thought all those word problems in grammar school were a waste of time.)

For assistance on playground safety, please call the National Program for Playground Safety at 1-800-554-PLAY (7529). Or check online at *www.playgroundsafety.org*.

The National Program for Playground Safety advises playgrounds to be:

S: *Supervisable:* Equipment is designed so you can see me while I play.

A: *Age appropriate:* Equipment is developed for specific ages. (4 months–2 years old), (2–5), (5–12)

F: *Falls to surfaces:* Suitable for me to fall on

E: *Equipment and surfacing are well maintained:* So I will not get severely injured and I can do what I do best—PLAY!!

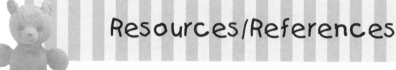

Resources/References

Car Seat Safety

If you have any questions about recalls or car safety you can check the Web site for the **National Highway Traffic Safety Administration** at *www.NHTSA.dot.gov.*

To find a certified technician to inspect the installation of your car seat go to *www.seatcheck.org* or call 1-866-SEAT-CHECK.

Playground Safety

For assistance on playground safety please call the **National Program for Playground Safety** at 1-800-554-PLAY (7529) or check online at *www.playgroundsafety.org.*

Product Safety

For questions regarding recalls and safety, contact the U.S. Consumer Product Safety Commission at *www.CPSC.gov*; toll-free hotline: 800-638-2772.

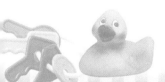

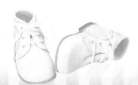

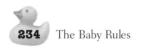

The Web site for all recalls by all agencies: *www.recalls.gov*.

National SAFE KIDS Campaign, *www.safekids.org*.

Pediatric Information and Vaccine Safety

American Academy of Pediatrics, *www.AAP.org*.

For vaccine questions, contact the **Vaccine Education Center** at The Children's Hospital of Philadelphia at *www.vaccine.chop.edu*.

Poisoning Information

The **National Lead Information Center,** 1-800-421-LEAD (424-5323) or contact the EPA Web site *www.epa.gov/led*.

Drinking water hotline—1-800-426-4791 or *www.epa.gov/safewater/hotline*.

National toll-free number for **Poison Control Centers:** 800-222-1222. You can call this number anytime from anywhere in the U.S., and your call will be automatically routed to the poison center nearest you.

Garden and Hearth.com—"Poisonous Plants."

American Association of Poison Control Centers—*AAPCC.org*

National Capital Poison Center—*www.poison.org*

Breastfeeding

For breastfeeding information contact: La Leche League International, 1400 N. Meacham Rd., Schaumburg, IL 60173-4808, (847) 519-7730. To find a local LLL Group, look for the listing for your state, province, or country on the LLLI Web site *www.lalecheleague.org;* or call 800-LA LECHE.

Anne Smith—BA, IBCLC, RLC, international board-certified lactation consultant, *www.breastfeedingbasics.com.*

Rosenthal, Sara, M. *The Breastfeeding Answer Book.* Lincolnwood: Lowell House, 2000.

La Leche League International. *The Womanly Art of Breastfeeding.* New York: Plume, 1997.

For breastfeeding accessories and pumps, go to *www.medela.com* or call 1-800-tell you.

Formula Information

Similac.com
Enfamil.com

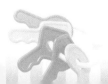
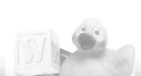

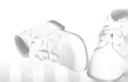

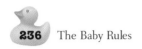

References

Breastmilk Storage Information: Pardou, A. "Human milk banking: Influence of storage processes and of bacterial contamination on some milk constituents." *Biol Neonate* 1994; 65:302-309.

Parenting Concerns: *The New Parents Guide—The New Parents Guide.com*—"Cloth vs. Disposable Diapers," "Is My Baby Teething?"

Pediatric Information: Bonnie Offit, M.D., Kids First—Haverford, Pennsylvania.

Psychological and Developmental Information: Alice Honig, Ph.D., professor emeritus of child development, Syracuse University, past president of the International Association for Infant Mental Health.

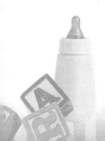
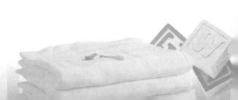

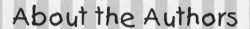

About the Authors

Jamie Schaefer-Wilson began her television career as an associate producer at "The Oprah Winfrey Show," where she learned the foundation for her trade from 1991 until 1993. She moved on to become an associate producer with the "Bertice Berry" show and then a producer at "The Gordon Elliott Show." At "The Gordon Elliott Show," she met coworker, fellow producer (and coauthor of *The Baby Rules*), Jo Anne Germinario. Jamie also worked as part of the media team for The Points of Light Foundation. There she produced a teleconference featuring General Colin Powell and then First Lady and now Senator Hillary Clinton, launching the Summit about the future of America's Children.

She was reunited with Jo Anne at the Sally Jessy Raphael show, where she worked as a senior producer and supervising producer. She married her husband, Steven Wilson, in June of 1999, and in August of 2000, Jamie found out she was pregnant. Jo Anne found out she was expecting, too, about one month later. The two women worked together, sharing an office with desks

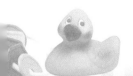

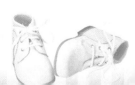

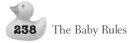

across from each other, while expecting their babies just a few weeks apart.

Jamie's daughter Cydney Rachel Wilson was born on March 28, 2001, and Cydney began her career as a teacher to her mommy almost immediately.

When "The Sally Show" ended, Jamie decided to devote her efforts to writing *The Baby Rules*.

Jo Anne Germinario began her television career as a news associate in 1989 at CNBC before the network was even on the air. After the launch of CNBC, she took a job with Geraldo Rivera. Jo Anne left "Geraldo" as an associate producer four years later and accepted a position as a producer for "The Gordon Elliott Show," where she met Jamie. Two years later, Jo Anne left the show to work as a producer for the newly created NBC show, "In Person with Maureen O'Boyle."

After the cancellation of "In Person," Jo Anne took some time off to get married to her husband, Anthony. After being called on a daily basis by Jamie offering a position at "The Sally Show," Jo Anne finally gave in and returned to her career as working mother once again. During her first year as a producer at "The Sally Show," Jo Anne gave birth to her son Anthony. She continued as a producer for one more year before being promoted to senior producer. Nine months later, Jo Anne found out that she and Jamie were both pregnant and expecting one month apart. They shared a one-of-a-kind experience, producing babies and talk shows at the same time, sharing an office, careers, pregnancies and friendship.

Jo Anne's daughter Michelle Maria Germinario was born on May 4, 2001.